PRAISE FOR

overcoming opioid addiction

"Outlines a commonsense solution to opioid dependency . . . a worthy read in a time when the stakes of opioid addiction are high."

—Booklist

"A desperately needed, science-based solution to the nation's worst-ever drug crisis."

    —Herbert D. Kleber, MD, founder of the Drug Dependence Unit, Yale University, and Division of Substance Abuse, Columbia University

"A must-read. Compassionate, readable, and scientifically sound, this is the first book I've seen that covers opioid addiction comprehensively and accurately. Dr. Bisaga masterfully reviews what caused the epidemic, the latest research on how to treat opioid use disorders, and how families and loved ones can effectively support those who are suffering. In the chaotic confusion in the media and elsewhere about how to solve this crisis, *Overcoming Opioid Addiction* presents both a clear path forward and the evidence to support it."

    —Omar Manejwala, MD, Chief Medical Officer, Catasys, and author of *Craving: Why We Can't Seem to Get Enough*

"*Overcoming Opioid Addiction* is an accessible, practical, comprehensive guide for health care providers, patients, and families. A great go-to source of information on all things opioids—I'm recommending it to my patients!"

    —Anna Lembke, MD, Chief of Addiction Medicine at Stanford University School of Medicine and author of *Drug Dealer, MD: How Doctors Were Duped, Patients Got Hooked, and Why It's So Hard to Stop*

overcoming opioid addiction

overcoming opioid addiction

The AUTHORITATIVE MEDICAL GUIDE for PATIENTS, FAMILIES, DOCTORS, and THERAPISTS

ADAM BISAGA, MD

with KAREN CHERNYAEV

Foreword by A. Thomas McLellan, PhD

THE EXPERIMENT

NEW YORK

The Experiment, LLC
220 East 23rd Street, Suite 600
New York, NY 10010-4658
theexperimentpublishing.com

Many of the designations used by manufacturers and sellers to distinguish their products are claimed as trademarks. Where those designations appear in this book and The Experiment was aware of a trademark claim, the designations have been capitalized.

The Experiment's books are available at special discounts when purchased in bulk for premiums and sales promotions as well as for fund-raising or educational use. For details, contact us at info@ theexperimentpublishing.com.

Library of Congress Cataloging-in-Publication Data

Names: Bisaga, Adam, 1963- author. | Chernyaev, Karen, 1961- author.
Title: Overcoming opioid addiction : the authoritative medical guide for
    patients, families, doctors, and therapists / Adam Bisaga, MD, with Karen
    Chernyaev.
Description: New York : The Experiment, 2018. | Includes bibliographical
    references.
Identifiers: LCCN 2018006152 (print) | LCCN 2018009242 (ebook) | ISBN
    9781615194599 (Ebook) | ISBN 9781615194582 (pbk.)
Subjects: LCSH: Opioid abuse--Treatment--United States.
Classification: LCC RC568.O45 (ebook) | LCC RC568.O45 B57 2018 (print) | DDC
    362.29/3--dc23
LC record available at https://lccn.loc.gov/2018006152

ISBN 978-1-61519-458-2
Ebook ISBN 978-1-61519-459-9

Cover design by Sarah Smith
Text design and illustration on p. 169 by Sophie Appel

Manufactured in the United States of America

First printing May 2018

10 9 8 7 6 5 4 3 2

*This book is dedicated to all the patients
I have had the privilege to work with.*

AN IMPORTANT NOTE TO READERS

This book contains the opinions and ideas of its authors. It is intended to provide helpful and informative material on the subjects addressed in the book. The book is not intended to be a substitute for professional medical advice, diagnosis, or treatment. Always seek the advice of a physician or other qualified health provider with any questions you may have regarding a medical condition. Do not disregard professional medical advice or delay in seeking it because of something you have read here.

The authors and publisher are providing this book and its contents on an "as is" basis and make no representations or warranties of any kind with respect to this book or its contents. The authors and publisher disclaim all such representations and warranties, including for example warranties of merchantability and educational or medical advice for a particular purpose. The authors and publisher specifically disclaim all responsibility for any liability, loss, or risk—personal or otherwise—that is incurred as a consequence, directly or indirectly, of the use and application of any of the contents of this book.

•

The stories in this book are true or composites of several cases. In most of the stories, names and other identifying information have been changed to protect anonymity. Any likeness to actual persons, either living or dead, is strictly coincidental.

Individuals with drug use disorders deserve nothing less than ethical and science-based standards of care that are available similar to the standards used in treatment of other chronic diseases.

—UNODC/WHO International Standards for the
Treatment of Drug Use Disorders, 2016

CONTENTS

Part 4: For Patients: What to Expect in Treatment and Beyond

FOREWORD

By A. Thomas McLellan, PhD

As the United States copes with the extraordinary health and social costs of our latest opioid addiction crisis, this solutions-oriented book—*Overcoming Opioid Addiction*—is particularly welcome. For those suffering from an opioid use disorder, their families, and the clinicians who treat them, Dr. Bisaga offers the most advanced, science-based methods for diagnosing, treating, and managing opioid addiction. As the book makes clear, even serious opioid addictions can be overcome. With comprehensive, continuing care full recovery is now an expectable result. The rationale and methods to achieve this goal are amply detailed in the book, and I can only hope all physicians and all families adopt the principles and practices Dr. Bisaga sets forth.

But there is a broader social context to the current addiction crisis that is also addressed by this book. Dr Bisaga shows why and how our country must get past our outdated and largely incorrect conceptions about addiction, substantially revise our antiquated set of addiction treatment programs, and fully integrate addiction prevention, early intervention, and treatment into mainstream healthcare—if we truly wish to overcome opioid (and other) addictions. In this regard, I do have some historical and conceptual comments that I hope will amplify the position Dr. Bisaga has taken.

Historically, addiction to alcohol and other drugs has been conceptualized as a sign of weak character, a personality disorder, or a habitual series of bad personal choices. This is easy to understand. Cardinal features of all addictions include failure to carry out normal adult role functions because of cravings for and uncontrolled use of alcohol or other drugs. For many seriously affected patients, lying, stealing, and negligent, dangerous acts (e.g. drunk driving) are all too common behavioral effects of the addiction. It's understandable then, why addictions have been stigmatized, and why they have been considered public safety problems to be dealt with through laws and punishments—rather than personal health problems better addressed through prevention, early intervention, and medical management.

For these reasons, since the late 1960s, virtually all available treatments for addiction have been provided by "addiction treatment programs" whose focus was on correcting the behavioral and character problems so typical among the seriously addicted. This was accomplished, usually by first treating the physical withdrawal and craving symptoms that were thought to fuel relapse; and then confronting the dishonesty and impulsive character traits that were thought to underlie an "addictive personality." Who better to lead this effort than peer counselors who were themselves modeling a new "recovery" lifestyle emphasizing personal honesty, social responsibility, and abstinence from all substance use. Under this conceptual framework and care delivery model, there was little need for physicians, medications, information systems, professional therapies, or most of the prominent features of modern healthcare.

So, it should not be surprising that the administration, regulation, and financing of the addiction treatment system occurred *outside* the mainstream healthcare system; or that addiction treatment was organized and financed primarily as an acute care system. The prevailing concept of addiction as a character or personality disorder did not fit well within the mainstream healthcare systems of the day, and physicians were neither trained for, nor particularly eager to accept patients with addictive disorders. A new system was purposely designed and financed to be separate from the rest of healthcare. Over the ensuing decades, as healthcare spending became an increasingly important issue within the private sector, employers made special efforts to reduce employee healthcare benefits for addiction treatment by purchasing "carved-out" insurance for addiction treatment, typically under the auspices of separate "behavioral health managed care organizations." By 2000, most addiction treatment was purchased with government funding (primarily state block grant and Medicaid dollars) and private insurance accounted for less than 12% of all care episodes.

There are two important but seldom acknowledged implications of this planned, purposeful segregation of addiction treatment. First, most major healthcare organizations eliminated addiction treatment. In turn, the great majority of medical, nursing, and pharmacy schools eliminated addiction education/training. Meanwhile, in mainstream healthcare, pharmaceutical benefits from private insurance packages fostered development of new medications with the promise of cheaper and more effective treatments; and there was a growing consumer movement—epitomized by those affected by HIV/AIDS—demanding more access and better treatments. These forces were never present in the addiction field, in part because the condition was so stigmatized that consumers felt unable to demand their rights. Because addiction was not accepted as an illness, medications were considered inappropriate by some providers, unnecessary by many state Medicaid systems, and clearly not profitable by most pharmaceutical companies. Drug counselors became the major professional group in the addiction field and group counseling became the most prevalent—often the only—available component of care. The result is that the approach and the content of addiction treatment has changed very little from its inception in the late 1960s until today. The remarkable advances in treating other diseases spurred by medical and pharmaceutical research and the consumer movement simply did not occur in the segregated addiction treatment system.

The critical, system-level point conveyed in this excellent book is that, as designed and constructed, the current addiction treatment system not only does not—it *cannot* provide the personalized care, management, and professionalism necessary to overcome opioid addiction. Dr. Bisaga's clinical guidelines for treating people with opioid or other addictions are, counterintuitively, more relevant and more achievable within today's primary care practices—though that would be news to most primary care physicians—than in most "traditional," non-medical addiction treatment programs. The clinical procedures described in this book offer an excellent basis for improving care for anybody with an opioid use disorder. But *overcoming opioid addiction* in this country will require addiction education in medical and nursing schools;

addiction treatment coverage at parity in healthcare insurance; and addiction prevention, early intervention, and treatment integrated throughout mainstream healthcare systems.

Put differently, without the transformation of concept, organization, financing, and management methods, addiction treatment is not likely to improve—regardless of scientific advances or public pressure. With an evidence-based rethinking of addiction as a chronic illness, training of primary care physicians, development of disease management protocols, adaptation of clinical information systems, benchmarking of standard measures of illness progression and patient improvement, and the development of personalized care monitoring and management practices, we will not only overcome opioid addiction—we will substantially improve the quality, effectiveness, and efficiency of mainstream healthcare.

A. Thomas McLellan, PhD
Emeritus, Department of Psychiatry,
Perelman School of Medicine, University of Pennsylvania
Former Deputy Director of the White House Office
of National Drug Control Policy

HOW TO USE THIS BOOK

Overcoming Opioid Addiction speaks to many audiences, and so I've divided it into four major sections: Part 1 covers general information about the epidemic, opioids, and addiction. Part 2 informs health-care professionals about expanding treatment of opioid use disorder (OUD) into existing medical settings and covers the intricacies of prescribing medication to people with OUD. Part 3 arms family members with vital information about how to live with an addicted loved one and coax them into getting help. It also describes what effective treatment looks like and how to go about finding it. Part 4 speaks directly to addicted individuals, or those who suffer from OUD and are in or contemplating treatment and recovery.

Regardless of the book's architecture, I encourage you to read the book in its entirety, even if you identify with only one of the audiences. You will comprehend the epidemic from various perspectives and encounter points of view you had not considered. Family members, for example, can make the most of this book by reading Part 2 for better insight into how opioids and the medications used to treat people work. Knowing at least some background information puts you in a better position to confidently ask important questions when seeking treatment for a loved one. Likewise, by reading Part 4, family members can learn a great deal about what it is like for their loved one to stop using painkillers or heroin. Professionals who do not normally work with patients addicted to opioids will find Parts 3 and 4 interesting and valuable as they may contemplate participating in the changing landscape of addiction treatment.

INTRODUCTION

In June 2016, delegates at an American Medical Association meeting boldly advocated that physicians should no longer monitor pain as a "fifth vital sign." The announcement echoed far and wide, throughout hospital hallways, pain clinics, treatment centers, households, homeless shelters, morgues, and law enforcement and legal entities, creating pause for such thoughts as *What if it had never happened?*

People in all of these settings had already felt the blows from measuring pain as a fifth vital sign, a practice much of the nation's medical community has adhered to for the past two decades. Although pain was relatively new addition to the four standard vitals of pulse, blood pressure, temperature, and respiration, the simple act of attempting to measure it has had an unprecedented impact: It inadvertently jump-started and helped carry to fruition what the president has declared a public health emergency and America's worst drug crisis ever—the epidemic of deaths related to opioid use, often called the opioid epidemic.

At its heart, the opioid epidemic seeks to destroy individuals who get addicted to the powerful substance. Many people change over the course of a few months, their one-track mind homing in on their next fix. Depending on the severity of the addiction, the consequences can range from mild to astronomical, affecting users physically, socially, emotionally, mentally, and even spiritually. Some lose homes and jobs and their families' trust. Families are thrown into a whirlwind of confusion as fear, lies, deceit, secrets, and arguments consume daily life. Personalities change as everyone struggles to deal with their new family dynamic. Attempts to control the drug use are futile and answers nowhere in sight. When it gets bad enough, families have no choice but to disown their loved one. They are not, it seems, able to do anything to help.

The epidemic is doing far more. It overtakes entire communities. Even children are not immune. A growing number of "opioid orphans," children who have lost their parents to regular opioid use or overdose, are overcrowding the foster care system. Parents overdose while parked in a shopping mall lot, their kindergartener forced to call 911 and explain that his dad's lips are turning blue. A librarian calmly calls 911 and matter-of-factly asks for paramedics to deliver naloxone, an overdose antidote, to the children's section, where a man is suspected of overdosing. Instead of dreaming about proms and college life, a once lively and engaged high schooler is now nodding off in class and at the dinner table.

Scared and ever confused about what to do, families put their lives on hold. When they finally get their loved one into residential treatment, sometimes depleting their life savings, they feel relief for the first time in years. Then they discover that treatment is just the beginning, not a cure-all. And so they walk on eggshells, knowing full well the statistics on the potential for relapse to today's plentiful opioids.

Yet there are success stories—stories of people who overcome the powerful lure of heroin and other opioids. These stories don't tend to make it into the daily news, but they exist. Like Michael, who went from standing on his apartment ledge to studying to become a drug counselor. Or Nicole, who found help and is now raising her toddler.

There is a way out. The pages of this book look not only at the epidemic but at what you can do to help a loved one, a patient, or an employee stop the madness. I offer a solution, a solid plan to help addicted individuals, families, and communities sort through what's happening, buy into a realistic perspective, and develop a set of priorities to lift everyone involved out of the chaos. This solution, firmly grounded in science as well as traditional approaches that demonstrate evidence-based merit, recognizes that opioid addiction is a physiologically based disorder whose long-term management requires appropriate medication administered within an enlightened and supportive social and professional network.

The Best of Intentions

The crisis started with the best of intentions. Those suffering from chronic pain had long been seen as being undertreated, primarily because physicians were reluctant to prescribe opioid painkillers for fear that their patients would develop a dependence on the highly soothing and addictive drugs. When powerful opioids became available for prescribing in the late 1990s, cautious physicians were reassured with a letter originally published in 1980 that claimed only a tiny percentage of patients actually became addicted to opioid painkillers. Drug companies, but also thought leaders, launched a campaign to de-stigmatize opioids as a strategy to manage chronic pain and the floodgates opened.

Fast-forward to 2015, when Americans were consuming an alarming 80 percent of the world's oxycodone and hydrocodone opioid painkillers (think: OxyContin and Vicodin) and 30 percent of all prescribed painkillers, even though Americans make up less than 5 percent of the world's population. For the first time ever, drug overdose became the leading cause of accidental death in the United States. In 2016, drug overdoses caused US life expectancy to fall for the second year in a row, a rare occurrence. Add to that a proliferation of powerful illicit opioids, not only heroin produced from poppies but also fentanyl and other deadly opioids made from scratch in laboratories. Over the past few years, heroin and synthetic opioids have overtaken painkillers as the drugs of choice for opioid users young and old, whether suffering from chronic pain or not.

Despite what some people believe, chronic pain and opioid addiction are not synonymous. Not everyone who has chronic pain and takes painkillers is addicted to opioids, and not everyone who takes painkillers has chronic pain. Nonmedical use of painkillers is now in many ways a bigger problem than medical use, with about 75 percent of opioid users introduced to the pills not by doctors but by friends and family who innocently offer a leftover pill to another in need. And so the real culprit is not always pain but the never-ending supply of painkillers—real and counterfeit—in circulation.

The national escalation of opioid use is mirrored in individual lives. As chronic pain patients, for example, adjust to their prescribed dosage, many need a stronger dose to alleviate their symptoms. Prescriptions, by definition, have set limits. Even refills are only for a certain number of pills. Addicted patients who cannot get their doctor to increase the dosage do what any addicted person would do. They get creative by filling prescriptions at several pharmacies (pharmacy hopping); stealing from the medicine cabinets of friends, neighbors, and family; buying pills from drug dealers or online; and finally turning to street drugs, namely heroin and its more lethal sister, fentanyl. As opioid users' tolerance grows, so does their need for a more potent fix. And so new and more powerful drug combinations with such names as "gray death" hit the market.

An Epidemic of Overdoses

Much more than a story of medical efforts to treat pain going south, the opioid epidemic is a perfect storm of many factors: Expert marketing, misinterpreted research, misguided youths, Big Pharma, the expansion of pill mills, and an eruption of home drug labs, drug cells, and cartels have all contributed to the problem, each seeming to appear onstage at just the right time, almost as if on cue. But what's most striking and alarming about the opioid epidemic is that, unlike other drug crises, overdose is intrinsic to it—deadly overdoses are occurring at unprecedented rates. A higher percentage of opioid users are dying today because the drugs they use are more dangerous than ever. Many of these deaths, for reasons we'll cover in this book, occur posttreatment. The repercussions of these untimely and unnecessary deaths linger with family members left to mourn their losses and wonder how on earth—in this day and age of advanced medicine, improved survival rates for most other disorders, tactical drug prevention campaigns, and trained treatment professionals—something fueled at its roots by compassion could go so wrong so quickly.

Opioids and opiates, a class of drugs that includes morphine, heroin, oxycodone (Percocet, OxyContin), and hydrocodone (Vicodin), have been around for centuries in one form or another. Their allure is nestled in the fact that they take away pain—physical, emotional, and mental. Their wrath is apparent in withdrawal, when feeling returns with a vengeance. Opioids create "junkies," people who need a daily fix, out of at least 20 to 25 percent of those who use them. Painkillers, whether for medical use or not, are often a gateway drug to heroin. And heroin, which is no stranger to America, is not going away anytime soon. For those interested in turning a quick profit, heroin is a model commodity, generally easy to process and transport and with a ready market. It is part of the legacy of many veterans returning from Afghanistan and Vietnam, and it played a large role in the counterculture of the sixties. But today's opioid crisis offers several alarming new twists. Heroin is purer and more potent, although still subject to being laced with deadly additives. New varieties of opioids are getting stronger and stronger. Use is widespread, and treatment availability and reach are dismal.

Opioid Use Disorder and Treatment

The key driver of the overdose epidemic is not just the drugs and the people who use them but how the human body reacts to opioids. The problem is often the underlying opioid use disorder (OUD). Only proper treatment of the disorder can effectively reduce the growing number of overdose deaths, yet more than twenty years into the epidemic, only one in five of the 2.4 million Americans with OUD received treatment, and less than half of them received effective, *evidence-based* treatment. Millions of Americans suffering from OUD, along with their pained family members, do not know that successful, evidence-based approaches specific to treating OUD exist. They do not know what to ask for or what to look for in terms of treatment. They do not understand that they have options. And so every day in this country, more than one hundred people die from opioid overdose, many of them posttreatment.

It is often said that drug addiction is an equal opportunity destroyer, knowing no boundaries when it comes to age, gender, race, or income. Never has this been truer than with opioids, whose reach extends beyond inner-city neighborhoods, affecting in large numbers white children in suburban households, middle-aged men in rural America, and retirees in senior housing facilities. Yet, as if to add insult to injury, some professionals are still arguing over the "right" approach to treating this condition.

Among addictions, OUD is a different animal, in part because of the dangerous level of tolerance to the drug an individual can develop, to the point where, in some respects, not using becomes more dangerous than using. It is a rare day when Columbia University addiction research psychiatrists proclaim that it is safer to continue to abuse heroin or prescription painkillers than it is to receive the treatment offered at most facilities in this country today. But as of this writing, the day has come. In fact, I would argue that it is now unethical for professionals to refer OUD patients to more than half of the treatment facilities in this country.

The Solution

Medication-assisted treatment (MAT), which combines medication and behavioral therapy, is a model of treatment created specifically for people addicted to opioids. The methods are tried and true. As of this writing, only a small percentage of those who need help have access to MAT. Most enter traditional treatment clinics unequipped or unwilling to deliver treatment with medication because it does not fit their definition of sobriety. Once released from traditional treatment, up to 90 percent of patients who do not receive medication relapse within the first three months. Many will overdose, as their detoxified bodies are unable to handle even a fraction of the amount of the drug they formerly consumed. Once detoxed, patients lose their tolerance for the drug. They are, in effect, newbies to opioids.

Death by opioid overdose is preventable. Yet the solution to the opioid crisis is complicated and manifold. It involves public education, community outreach, changing the way physicians approach the treatment of pain, and access to evidence-based addiction treatment and recovery services. Unlike with previous epidemics, there is no illusion that we can stall its progress by incarcerating people. We understand that connecting patients with proper treatment is what works. Proper treatment is available to us. We know what works. But what works is contrary to tradition, and so acceptance is painfully slow. Each day wasted clinging to a traditional method that is clearly inadequate for treating OUD is another day where a hundred people die, chasing a high they will never again find and seeking relief to the pain their bodies will never heal from. At least, not while under the spell of opioids.

This book is for you—opioid users seeking recovery, as well as the families, doctors, treatment providers, community leaders, and policy makers who want to learn how to help those who have fallen into the hell of opioid addiction. I include all that I have learned over the past two decades of working with opioid-addicted patients and their families, merging what science and my patients have taught me about treating OUD. Beyond the story of how opioids became such an issue, you will find important information about the drugs and learn the physiology behind not only addiction but the unique way in which opioids overtake the brain. Family members will learn how to reverse an overdose, assist a loved one through withdrawal, how to care for a pregnant woman with the disorder and her baby, and how to live with them while gently coaxing them into treatment and then supporting their recovery. Opioid users will read about what to expect in treatment and beyond, the challenges as well as the joys. Most important, you will comprehend that there is a solution. It is not traditional, and it is not newfangled. It is not failure-proof, either. But it is evidence based and far more effective for OUD than traditional treatment is. It can save lives and communities, and there is a good chance it can help you, your family, or your patients.

First and foremost, the opioid crisis is about people. Not just people who use drugs, but the people whose lives they touch.

PART 1

An Epidemic Like Never Before

CHAPTER 1

Medical Panacea
or National Nightmare?

In **eastern Ohio,** a police officer has just finished apprehending two individuals in possession of illegal drugs when fellow officers point out that his uniform is dusted slightly with the confiscated white powder. Using his bare fingertips, he instinctively and casually brushes it off. Within seconds, this healthy, muscular man in his prime drops to the ground. His skin has absorbed the drug, and he instantly overdoses. After receiving four doses of naloxone—the opioid overdose reversal medication—he survives, but not without kicking himself for not remembering his first-responder training. Even a minuscule dosage of fentanyl is potent enough to kill a newbie to opioid use. The body simply cannot handle it.

Fentanyl, an opioid similar to morphine but fifty to a hundred times more potent, is part and parcel of the current opioid crisis, one of the longest and most deadly drug epidemics in US history. Fentanyl attracts heroin users looking for a higher high, or something with more bang for their buck. The body that has developed a tolerance for opioids demands more, and seasoned opioid users will take fentanyl even if they see someone overdose from it right before their eyes. In a drug-seeking state, nothing is more important, and the high seems worth the risk.

Leading the Nation

Over the past twenty-some years, using opioids for nonmedical purposes has been credited with a long list of national records:

- Beginning in 2015, drug overdose became the leading cause of accidental death.

- In 2016, the number of deaths involving opioids surpassed the number of deaths from breast cancer.

- Reported fatal overdoses for all drugs reached 63,600 in 2016, up 20 percent from 2015; 66 percent involved opioids.

- More than 42,000 died from opioid overdose in 2016 (up 28 percent over 2015).

- Between 2013 and 2016, deaths from fentanyl rose by 540 percent.

- In 2009, the number of people entering treatment for opioid use disorder was six times great than in 1999, increasing by more than 11 percent every year.

- In 2015, 122,000 adolescents were addicted to prescription painkillers, and a total of 276,000 used the drugs for nonmedical purposes.

- Between 1999 and 2010, 48,000 women died of prescription painkiller overdose.

The story of the officer is not unusual. It has happened elsewhere, even after, in the summer of 2016, the Drug Enforcement Agency issued a warning to all first responders regarding exposure to the powerful narcotics. It is a small yet significant example of the far-reaching collateral damage of today's opioid epidemic, where the norm is for law enforcement, weighed down in hazmat suits, to undergo an expensive and laborious decontamination process after confiscating even small amounts of opioids. Clearly, the epidemic affects more than just those using opioids.

In Towns Hardest Hit

In towns hardest hit, including communities in Ohio, Kentucky, West Virginia, and New Hampshire, parents hesitate to take their kids to the park, where they're likely to witness an overdose or two, and 911 call attendants hear frantic pleas for help from children whose parents have overdosed. Paramedics can spend the majority of their shifts administering naloxone (brand name Narcan) to overdose victims. The overdose reversal medication saves lives but is criticized for "encouraging" high-risk use. Some people make sure to use the buddy system when shooting up, knowing if they overdose, their friend will phone for naloxone.

Employers struggle to fill open positions, as only a handful of applicants can pass the drug test. Those who test positive for opioids and produce a prescription are cleared, even if they are injecting heroin on the side. The drug test does not calculate on moral grounds—it cannot differentiate between legal and illegal opioids. By year's end, many new hires quit, get fired, or die from overdose. And, like the Ohio police officer, law enforcement and other first responders must now confront a new, more ethereal weapon—exposure to such opioids as fentanyl.

And so must toddlers who inadvertently get into Mom's or Dad's stash. Mistaking it for candy or curious about how it tastes, they ingest amounts that would kill an adult. In 2015, the Centers for Disease Control and Prevention reported that 87 children died that year from accidental exposure to opioids, up from 16 in 1999.

This is the new normal. The stories are endless, so much so that the term *opioid*, once reserved mostly for scientific use, has now become a household word, splashed across newspaper headlines on a daily basis. So, what are opioids? And why, after more than twenty years, is the opioid crisis still so out of hand?

Poppy: The Joy Plant

Perhaps no other plant in the world has been the source of so much joy and grief all at the same time as the poppy. In some countries, it's illegal to plant it. In others, fields of it grow free and wild. In still others, it makes up a significant percentage of the gross national product. It's been the cause of war, the subject of poems, a medical panacea, and its seeds the filling of delicious breads and pastries. A large field of it puts Dorothy and her entourage to sleep when approaching Oz. It is California's state flower and is featured on the emblem of London's Royal College of Anaesthetists.

The poppy is one of the most important medicinal plants known to humankind. It is a welcome source of pain relief for cancer patients in hospice and under palliative care. Most surgeons and oncologists rely on it for their patients. It can relieve an intractable cough, treat disorders of the gut, instantly lift depression or anxiety, and even quell psychosis. It also produces unmatched euphoria and spectacular dreams, which is why some people find it a great source of joy, at least initially, and have done so since ancient times. The poppy has been cultivated since the Neolithic period. The Sumerians tagged it "the joy plant."

The poppy plant seems innocent enough. In fact, just looking at it can make you happy. Its pretty petals create a fantastic display of red, yellow, purple, or blue. But the center of the flower—its fruit, or the pod—is what gets everyone's serious attention. When the fruit first ripens, it contains a milky and gooey sap (latex). Incising the green pod causes the sap to ooze out, and, when left to dry, the sap becomes a solid brown substance known as raw opium. Opium is one of nature's most powerful soporific agents. In small, sporadic doses, it relieves many unpleasant symptoms and makes its users happy. In large doses, it's poisonous. Chronic use can lead to misery.

Once harvested, dried, molded, and cooked, opium can be smoked in a pipe (recall the smoke-filled opium dens in the western United States in the late 1800s), drunk as a tea, dissolved and injected, taken as a suppository, or eaten whole by those who can stomach its bitter, earthy flavor. For variation, it's sometimes mixed with tobacco, a flower from a cannabis plant, or wine or rum. To this day, doctors prescribe opium tincture—made of opium, saffron, and high-proof alcohol—to treat diarrhea.

Opium can also be made more powerful. Morphine, used in medicine for analgesic (painkilling) purposes, is derived from opium and is ten times stronger (10 kilograms of opium produce 1–1.5 kg of morphine). In turn, 1 kilogram of morphine makes 1 kilogram of heroin, which is four times stronger than morphine when injected.

Most people are familiar with *opiate*, the term used to describe any drug directly derived from opium. These include morphine, codeine, hydrocodone, and heroin. The term *opioid* is more inclusive. It embraces all opium-based drugs (opiates), as well as those created in a laboratory to mimic opium by activating the same receptor sites in the brain. Most prescription painkillers currently on the market, including oxycodone (OxyContin), hydromorphone (Dilaudid), fentanyl, and methadone are synthesized. Synthesized opioids can be much stronger than opiates. Fentanyl, for example, is fifty to one hundred times more powerful than morphine.

Opiates

Natural alkaloids isolated from poppy resin (opium)
- Morphine
- Codeine
- Thebaine

Semi-synthetic substances derived from natural alkaloids

Drugs made from morphine
- Diacetylmorphine (heroin)
- Hydromorphone (Dilaudid, Exalgo)

Drugs made from Codeine
- Hydrocodone (used in combination tablets with acetaminophen (Vicodin, Norco, Lorcet) or with ibuprofen (Vicoprofen)

Drugs made from Thebaine
- Oxycodone (OxyContin, Roxicodone); sometimes used in combination with acetaminophen (Percocet)
- Oxymorphone (Opana)
- Buprenorphine (Buprenex, Probuphine, Subcolade); sometimes used in combination with naloxone (Suboxone, Zubsolv, Bunavail)

Synthetic Opioids

- Methadone (Dolophine, Methadose)
- Fentanyl (Sublimaze, Actiq, Subsys, Duragesic)
- Meperidine (Demerol)
- Pentazocine (Talwin)
- Butorphanol
- Tramadol (Ultram)
- Loperamide (Imodium)

Opium's Growing Assault

It seems that there is no limit to how much we can manipulate opium's potency. The current epidemic has brought out from the shadows drugs that existed but were never before intentionally consumed by humans, and these substances are literally enough to drop an elephant. A mere 2 milligrams of fentanyl, the weight of three grains of sugar, is considered lethal to an average-size person. The same amount of the fentanyl-like drug carfentanil, which is often synthesized with other opioids and really is used to tranquilize elephants, is one hundred times stronger.

Carfentanil's uses go beyond veterinary medicine. In scientific and military arenas, *carfentanil* is synonymous with "weapon." The substance is banned for use in battle under the Chemical Weapons Convention, although until recently it was produced and sold legally in China. Not everyone who takes carfentanil knows what they are taking. Some who are just trying to get their daily fix may unwittingly buy heroin laced with the potent tranquilizer. Unless they have developed an extremely high tolerance to opioids, they likely will not live to tell about it.

Such savagely strong drugs fill a gap in the market. They are cheaper than heroin and do not have to be smuggled into the United States from Mexico or Afghanistan. Clandestine laboratories create new illicit opioids sometimes on a monthly basis. With such names as MT-45, U-4, or U-47700, these drugs are many times stronger than morphine. Some of them are pressed to look identical to legally produced pharmaceutical medications, trademark symbol and all, duping buyers into believing that they know what they are getting.

These newer drugs make heroin look like child's play. But why would anyone intentionally consume a chemical weapon? And why would anyone produce such lethal drugs, knowing full well that the consumers will likely not be repeat customers?

For illegal drug producers, it is a gamble worth taking. Investment costs are minimal and the profits outrageous. A pill press and wholesale fentanyl precursors purchased, often legally, overseas can reap millions of dollars after being cooked up into a fentanyl powder and made into fake pills or fake heroin in a basement laboratory. And, just as there is no end to the potency of opioids, there seems to be no end to the number of people willing to self-destruct to get their next fix.

It's as if the country had a death wish. This is the power behind opioid addiction.

How Did We Get Here?

The connection between opium, opiates, and opioids is relative to our discussion—to understanding not just the terminology but also the channel through which opioids travel. Synthesized opioids are not just illegal substances but essential legal analgesics, some designed to help patients get through fierce and otherwise untreatable pain. Fentanyl, for example, is given to cancer patients in palliative care who no longer respond to tamer painkillers. These patients are at the end of life, trying to minimize excruciating pain. Morphine is commonly used during and after surgery, on the battlefield, and in hospice, when patients are thought to have six months or less to live. In these cases, addiction is usually the least of anyone's concerns. Treating pain and ensuring comfort are the primary objectives.

Painkillers are also prescribed for less serious acute pain—to take home after a root canal or when a broken wrist has been cast, for example. In these circumstances, many people can get by with an Advil or a Tylenol, so they place the Percocet in the medicine cabinet for a rainy day, close the door, and forget about it. Those with a lower pain threshold or who want to follow doctor's orders might decide to take the medicine as prescribed. A large percentage are overcome with nausea and swear off the stuff, or they feel they could take it or leave it. About one quarter of those who try it, however, enjoy it.

Eric is one such person.

Eric plays linebacker on his high school's varsity football team. He occasionally drinks alcohol and smokes pot, though not during football season. He lives for the game, and he knows that if he were caught using, even in a photograph, he'd be off the team. Rules are rules. And he has no problem abstaining.

His senior year, Eric gets injured during the second game and has to sit out the rest of the season. Suddenly, all he is living for is on hold. Eric gets a bit depressed thinking about everything he is missing out on. He is a good athlete and was hoping for a football scholarship for college. Now, he is fully aware that this will likely be his last year of organized team sports.

At the hospital, Eric is treated for a broken arm and gets a bottle of prescription painkillers to take home. He takes them as directed to relieve the soreness. The pills lift not only his pain but also his mood, and his prospects do not appear as dim anymore. After about a week, Eric's pain goes away, but he continues taking the pills to elevate his mood, as they make him feel great.

No longer on the practice field or lifting weights and otherwise training, Eric finds himself with a lot of free time. His best friends are busy playing sports, so he starts hanging out with friends who drink and smoke. These friends introduce him to Xanax, a sedative.

Eric's motivation for schoolwork dives and so do his grades. Now he is physically dependent: He has to take painkillers every day or he faces excruciating stomach and shoulder pain and is agitated, anxious, and cannot sleep. Eric calls the pharmacy for a refill, but his doctor does not renew the prescription. Eric starts buying pills from friends and then the black market. After a month, he runs out of money, so he sells his electronic devices and steals from his parents to support his habit. He isolates himself from friends and is often irritable and hard to be with. He is frequently seen arguing with his girlfriend.

After Eric takes a few pills, all of his many problems seem to vanish, and so he keeps using. His friends and coach (who sees him on game days—often with a vacant stare) are worried. The coach finally calls his parents, who stage an intervention and give him an ultimatum.

The Erics of the World

Most of the Erics of the world start taking painkillers as prescribed, and when their one- or two-week prescription runs out, they call to ask the doctor for more. (Usually at the original time of prescription, they are not told that they could get addicted, develop a physical dependence, and have their life destroyed by the medication—or they skip reading the pharmaceutical company's minuscule-font warnings in the package.) They complain that they are still in pain and could they please have a refill. The doctor has no way of knowing for sure how much pain they are in, exactly, as pain cannot be measured with a test. A doctor can go by experience, but experience dictates that everyone responds to pain differently. Most doctors have little to no schooling in how to recognize addiction, and, even for the trained eye, addiction can be hard to spot. Patients may claim that on a scale of 1 to 10, their pain level is an 8. And so they get a refill. But instead of taking one pill every four hours, they now take one pill every two hours. Their body seems to need it; they feel distressed without it.

Before long, these folks find themselves unable to think about anything but getting more painkillers. When the prescription runs out, they plead with an already suspicious doctor, visit more doctors, pharmacy hop, search internet forums, or maybe invade the "rainy day" medicine cabinets of friends and family. Even if they do get another refill, it's not enough. For those who are genetically predisposed to addiction, prescription medication use quickly—sometimes within a matter of a few months—turns to illicit drug use. Their body develops a tolerance to the drug so that to feel any kind of effect, they need more pills, must resort to more dangerous delivery methods (e.g., snorting or injecting), or seek something stronger. Buying pills off the street is expensive: One pill of OxyContin (30 milligrams) can cost $30, and many people need numerous pills per day. Heroin is cheaper. The same bang can be had for less than half the cost of a prescription pill. A fentanyl patch can cost up to $100. But what is sold on the streets isn't monitored or regulated, and the potential for taking a lethal dosage looms eternal.

A Temporary Solution Gone Mad

Opioid painkillers are meant to be a temporary solution. And I would add "for serious pain." In many patients, opioids stop being effective painkillers when used chronically, after several weeks to a few months. But the body can develop such a high tolerance to opioids that to stop using the accustomed amount is an experience akin to not eating. The body needs sustenance. Without it, the body craves and pursues its "nourishment."

Many of those who first try opioids aren't looking to get high. They want to relieve pain. But even when people start using opioids recreationally, for the drugs' euphoric and stimulating effect, eventually the opioids stop working, as is the nature of many mood-altering substances. As their bodies shore up a "natural defense system" against intoxicants, they must seek a higher dose or a stronger opioid and take it more frequently just to feel "normal."

In a seminal experiment conducted by Abraham Wikler in the 1950s—one that would nowadays be considered unethical—volunteers with a history of heroin use were given unlimited access to injectable morphine and allowed to "readdict" themselves while the researchers carefully observed the volunteers' behavior. Over the course of less than four months, one volunteer increased his morphine intake forty-six-fold, more by increasing the frequency of injections than by increasing each dosage. At the end, he was taking and tolerating enough morphine to kill five or more people who are naive to the drug. This rapid development of tolerance is not unique to opioids—it happens with cocaine, marijuana, and alcohol, too—but even the strongest alcohol (pure grain alcohol, at 190 proof) does not come close to the strength of today's opioids. A high dose of opioids can kill in a matter of minutes by shutting down breathing. The body's only defense against it is tolerance.

The means by which people enter the world of mood-altering drug use are many and go well beyond clinic doors: the overworked doctor with access to meds, the adolescent who wants to fit in, the father of three who just lost his job, and the young woman with a history of sexual trauma. Everyone has a story. How they sustain use also varies but usually involves illegal street drugs, of which there seems to be no limit. But there is at least one common denominator: Addicted people are like a moth to a flame. They keep going after their drug of choice even though they get burned. Addiction overrides self-preservation instincts.

The Road to Treatment

I've personally never met an opioid-addicted person who is proud of their behavior. They might be scarred by not only an armful of needle marks but also a great deal of shame and self-hatred. They know their behavior has ruined their lives and caused everyone they love grief. But they can't stop. Some try to quit on their own, but when deprived of opioids, the body lashes back with severe withdrawal symptoms, forcing a quick return to using. Those who still have a support system might find themselves in a medically supervised detoxification unit, which assuages symptoms, followed by treatment. Treatment should be everyone's best option. But opioid addiction is a different animal, and in some cases, treatment inadvertently does more harm than good.

Eric, for instance, reluctantly admits there is an issue with his current drug use. He is not entirely convinced he needs residential treatment, but at the behest of his community of loved ones and supporters, he agrees to go. Eric spends twenty-eight days in a residential treatment program that is covered by his health insurance, and his family breathes a sigh of relief that the most difficult part is behind them. They are hopeful that once the drug is out of Eric's system, he will be fine. His medically supervised detox with standard withdrawal medication leaves him feeling weak and sleeping poorly for a week but is far better than the torment he experienced stopping opioids on his own at home. Within a few days of arriving, he is put into treatment groups among others in recovery, learning about how to apply the Twelve Steps in daily life as well as the workings of Narcotics Anonymous (NA).

In treatment, Eric meets other young opioid users, some of them sentenced to treatment unwillingly with criminal justice oversight. After meetings, these kids talk a lot about drug use and share stories of how to get high. Eric hears about crushing and sniffing pills for greater effect and all about heroin—where to get it and how to use it. Some of the kids have plans to use again once their probation is over. Eric, however, is committed to abstinence. He leaves the treatment center with a relapse-prevention plan, recommendations to attend NA meetings, and instructions to use the skills he learned in treatment to deal with triggers and cravings.

Following treatment, Eric is connected with peers in the local recovery community. A sociable guy, Eric willingly attends NA meetings, where he enjoys the camaraderie and support. Drug-free, he feels good, if not a little unsure, but he feels he benefits from the program. After two months of regular attendance at NA meetings, life gets busier and he gradually tapers off. The treatment center calls him for a follow-up report. He mentions that he is doing well and agrees to stay in touch on the phone every three months, even though he is not as committed to the Twelve Step fellowship as he was in the past.

Life goes on, and Eric goes to college, though not on a sports scholarship as he had hoped. His first semester is stressful, but there is a lively partying scene. Problems go away on the weekend with drinking and smoking. He is not abstaining from all mood-altering drugs, but he is not using painkillers. One Saturday night, Eric gets drunk at a party. Someone pulls out a bottle of painkillers to share. At first, Eric doesn't pay any attention. After a few more beers, he lets his guard down and cherry-picks a painkiller. One pill, he decides, will not do any harm. He has an amazing experience, feels euphoric and invincible and ready to take on the challenge of college.

For several days afterward, Eric cannot seem to shrug off thoughts about his experience. He thinks about using again. Just entertaining those thoughts makes him excited, and he actively fantasizes about how good he will feel. Eric has not had these kinds of thoughts before. He recognizes that painkillers caused problems, yet he convinces himself that he knows now how to control their use. He surmises that he can use them sparingly so that the pills are helpful.

Eric's use gradually escalates, but he continues to think he is in control and that he won't repeat old mistakes and become addicted again. He knows the ropes now. At first, he takes painkillers recreationally every weekend, but soon it becomes a daily thing. Random thoughts of using preoccupy Eric and prevent him from shifting his attention elsewhere. After he swallows a pill, everything seems to be back to normal. He quickly develops a tolerance for opioids, and the number of pills he needs to feel "normal" is hard to come by. He remembers what he learned in rehab and starts crushing and sniffing his pills to enhance the effects. As he runs out of money, he buys heroin and starts sniffing it two or three times per day. Soon, he loses motivation, stops going to classes, and has to drop out on medical leave. His anxiety and depression escalate.

The Problem with Treatment

There are a lot of ways to look at Eric's relapse: He has no willpower, he is lazy, he does not care; he just wants to get high; he failed; he did not work his recovery program hard enough; he should have gone to more meetings; he should have been more forthright during the follow-up calls; or he should have told his parents and asked for help. Although any of the above might have some kernel of truth to it, I would wager that none is the real source of Eric's relapse. Eric was set up to fail, through bad advice from well-meaning friends and family and a largely outdated addiction treatment system that does not reflect the scientific progress made in addiction treatment over the past fifty years.

Eric, however, was lucky. He relapsed and did not die. But remember the police officer at the beginning of this chapter? He was not an opioid user. His body had zero tolerance for the drug, and he overdosed from simply touching fentanyl. People who detox and then abstain from opioids also have zero tolerance. If they relapse, there is no telling how much of what opioid they will consume. They might even think they can handle the amount they consumed before entering treatment and detoxing. If they unknowingly consume a counterfeit pill containing fentanyl or take more pills than their body can tolerate, they have not only relapsed but overdosed, sometimes fatally.

Relapses happen every day to people like Eric. With opioids, more than any other drug, relapse can be fatal, especially to a detoxified body. Eric's relapse was not inevitable, and the most tragic part of it is that he is not an isolated example. Eric did not know that there is another way of looking at his struggles other than the one he learned about in the program. He was not given a chance to try another approach to treatment, one that could have been more useful in the long term.

When someone in the family is using heroin, most people do not call a doctor trained in addiction medicine. They turn to family and friends who might have had a problem with addiction. They arrange to meet with a relative, say an uncle, who is an alcoholic in recovery and has been sober for twenty years. Sincerely wanting to help, he explains that he went to residential treatment followed by regular attendance at Alcoholics Anonymous (AA). He says he still goes to AA meetings weekly, is doing very well, and in fact loves his life in recovery. His advice is to go to detox, go to rehabilitation, and then go to a Twelve Step meeting every day for ninety days and then weekly afterward. And so the family escorts their loved one to a traditional treatment center.

The Twelve Step program is based on a set of spiritual principles and requires abstinence from all mood-altering substances. It has helped millions of people worldwide find a meaningful life in recovery since its inception in the 1930s. The program is based on the work of Bill Wilson, one of the founders of Alcoholics Anonymous, who wrote an inspired list of twelve steps that alcoholics need to take to achieve not only sobriety but a full life. The book *Alcoholics Anonymous* (affectionately known as the "Big Book") followed. Its stories of recovering people and explanations of how the steps work serve as the basic text of AA. The book helps alcoholics understand addiction and learn how to live without alcohol, or their drug of choice. The Big Book is influential, to say the least. It is handed out to every person who attends a Twelve Step program. Since 1939, it has sold more than thirty million copies, making it one of the world's best-selling books.

In the 1930s, there was no medical model for treating alcoholism. Alcoholics joined together in AA meetings, where they could admit to their addiction and tell their story. By sharing their experiences and wisdom, alcoholics helped one another overcome alcoholism. For many, this alone had an incredible healing effect. Before long, a set of principles derived from the experiences of Twelve Step groups started to be used as a *treatment* strategy—the Twelve Step program. Since the Twelve Step program is not a biological treatment, it did not require rigorous scientific testing or any formal approval. Eventually, providers began using the approach to treat addiction to substances other than alcohol, including opioids, again with little to no scientific testing.

When various medications to help reduce substance use became available, Twelve Step programs did not incorporate them into their traditional model of treatment. Rather, the two ways of treating addictions developed in parallel: a traditional drug-free approach and a medical approach that offers medication in addition to behavioral treatment. Both approaches were and still are useful in the treatment of alcoholism. For more than thirty years, however, scientific studies have shown that the Twelve Step program alone, even when combined with other intensive psychosocial interventions, does not serve most people with opioid addiction. Not in these days of carfentanil, gray death, and MT-45. Traditional treatment programming alone has not proven capable of responding to the unfolding epidemic of opioid overdose deaths. Yet the majority of treatment centers nationwide are built on this model for treating alcoholics. The overarching problem is that traditional treatment is not equipped to handle the changes in the brain associated with regular opioid use.

Fighting Fire with Fire

Opioid addiction, officially known as opioid use disorder (OUD), always begins with someone using opioids, either for pleasure or to relieve pain. Continued use of the drug by someone with a genetic risk for addiction changes normal activity in several regions of that person's brain. The presence of stressors in the environment accelerates and intensifies these changes. At a point, the brain begins to overreact to stress and stimuli associated with drug use. Two symptoms of this pathological response are the constant thinking about the drug and powerful urges to use. Meanwhile, the parts of the brain that would normally inhibit unwanted behaviors have become less effective in stopping impulses to use. This abnormal brain activity, a genuine physiological change, can persist even after months of abstinence.

The way to heal the disordered brain is to understand how the disorder develops and then create a medical strategy to counteract or reverse it. Health-care professionals look at the biological aspects of a disorder, treat it accordingly, educate patients about their disorder, and monitor those patients for the duration of the disorder. This is the medical model. The methodology is applied in all branches of medicine and, in this day and age, informed by science.

Science has proven that certain medications can stabilize abnormal responses that have developed in the brains of people with OUD. These medications—methadone, buprenorphine, and naltrexone—have been used medically for more than forty years. Methadone and buprenorphine, both opioids, were first used to treat pain, and naltrexone was developed to treat opioid addiction. Over the years, researchers tested these medications as OUD treatments. The Food and Drug Administration (FDA), a federal agency responsible for protecting public health, reviewed the results of these studies and determined that the three medications were safe and effective for the treatment of OUD. These government-sanctioned treatments are based on proven results. They are evidence based.

Copious studies have shown that each of these medications has unique benefits and limitations, may have side effects, may be misused, and may even be harmful, as is the case with many other medicines in use today. Not everyone will have a complete and sustained response, and some may have to try more than one medication more than once. But when the right medication is administered correctly, individuals show marked improvement: reduced thoughts about the drug and fewer and less powerful urges to use; improved mood and sleep; and an enhanced ability to think, plan, and resist impulses. All of these changes add up to protection against relapse.

The evidence-based approach to treating opioid addiction has success rates similar to treatments for many medical and psychiatric disorders, including diabetes, hypertension, or a recurrent major depressive disorder. Like these other disorders, OUD is chronic, and the affected person remains vulnerable to relapse for a long time. Because of this, people with OUD should be offered medical and psychosocial interventions over their life span, with intensity corresponding to the severity of symptoms. Each of the FDA-approved medications used to treat OUD works best in conjunction with psychosocial and behavioral therapies—including the Twelve Step program—to help patients achieve and maintain recovery. Yet in some people with mild OUD, therapy is not necessary. Medication by itself is enough to support complete and sustained remission of the disorder. In stark contrast to treatments for most other disorders, however, very few patients receive evidence-based treatment with medication for OUD.

The traditional attempt at a brief detoxification followed by a drug-free, or abstinence-based, approach has no evidence for effectively treating opioid addiction. In addition, this approach can be very dangerous. Detoxed patients who do not receive medication face an elevated risk of dying from an overdose if they relapse. Postdetox, the body can no longer tolerate the amount of opioids once consumed. You could call it death by detox. Sadly, too many of us have witnessed it on too many occasions.

More than one hundred individuals, many of them young adults, die of opioid overdoses every day. Some of them die after receiving traditional treatment, where using medications to assist in recovery-oriented treatment has no place. Treatment that includes medications is proven to be the best way to help a person addicted to opioids and reduce the number of deaths on a large scale. Yet resistance to change comes primarily from the people who have devoted their careers to helping addicted individuals—the ones who fully understand addiction as a disorder and a treatable one at that. They cling to an abstinence-based program and reject the use of medications, FDA approved or not, to help their opioid-addicted patients. This resistance is not based on a lack of evidence; rather, on a more spiritual than medical perspective that views using medication to recover as a step backward. Yet a doctor would never suggest that a diabetic not take insulin for spiritual reasons. Medication does not usually interfere with spiritual goals. The spiritual and medical can and do coexist in recovery.

Resistance to change in the addiction treatment field is based not only on tradition but also on a traditional problem: Most addiction treatment clinics do not have the funds for a medical wing, much less the medical staff needed to monitor and administer the medications. And so they continue to operate as they always have. Less than 10 percent of the approximately three thousand residential addiction treatment programs in this country have an addiction medical professional, a physician, or a nurse practitioner on staff. People with OUD who enter these doors do not have much of a chance against the lure of today's opioids, because these people need something that most programs cannot offer them. At present, medications are our best weapon against the opioid crisis.

The Bridge into Recovery

Traditional treatment professionals are not the only group opposed to giving addicted individuals medication to heal. The general public can be leery about doling out tax dollars for programs to help someone who does not contribute to society and breaks the law. The stigma around addiction has softened over the years, but it still exists in spades, especially when it

comes to hard-core drugs, such as heroin. It is safe to say th[
public is more interested in reading the sensationalized sto[
travails and demise of addicted individuals than they are in[
individual out of the mire. After reading this chapter, you may[
be convinced that most individuals addicted to opioids are m[_]victims
than criminals and that they spend more time suffering than enjoying a
high. If not, you might at least agree with what science has proven—that
addiction is a disorder that can be managed, like diabetes or hypertension,
and that it would be criminal not to provide medication to an individual
who needs it to survive.

Many politicians favor using medication to support behavioral treatment
efforts, although with some caveats. Former US congressman Tim Murphy
of Pennsylvania, a strong reformer of mental health legislation, talked about
medication as a bridge for opioid addicts, a bridge from addiction to recovery.
I would like to borrow that metaphor. Murphy advocated for a short bridge,
where opioid addicts walk off after a predetermined time period. But who
determines how long the bridge should be? Do we push people off at a certain
point? Do they jump? These are valid questions since, currently, the line to
get on the bridge is long, and it keeps getting longer.

The questions then become: How long do people with OUD *need* to
stay on their medication therapy? How much time and money will we spend
supporting them? Let me answer this with more questions: How long does a
person with high blood pressure stay on diuretics or calcium channel blockers?
How long does a diabetic stay on insulin? And who is paying for their care?

Medications have been shown to reduce overdose rates for opioid-
addicted individuals by more than 50 percent while those people are retained
in care. However, to be successful, most patients require long-term maintenance treatment with medications well beyond initial improvement. Continuing medication not only stops OUD symptoms, such as craving and
thoughts of using, but prevents these distressing symptoms from recurring.
The most effective treatments last years rather than months. For some, treatment may be lifelong. We do not know (yet) how to tell who will need lifelong
treatment versus short-term care. We cannot quantify the risk of relapse after

curtailed treatment, but it is not insubstantial. I know of no studies that demonstrate the benefit of premature cessation of maintenance medications for opioid addiction, but the opposite has been observed frequently. After medication is stopped, many patients, including those who have been stable for some time, will destabilize.

The decision regarding how long to keep someone on medication cannot be made in advance. The patient's progress must be evaluated and reevaluated. Someday, we will have even better medications or better methods of predicting who can come off when. But for now, giving patients a predetermined timeline at the start of treatment can be harmful. It sets up false expectations and even a sense of failure if the patient is not ready or able to taper by a given date. We do not determine duration of treatment up-front with cancer patients or people who have any other systemic chronic illnesses. Why should OUD patients be treated differently?

Swapping One Addiction for Another?

Opponents of long-term treatment based on the medical model criticize long-term use of medication as swapping one addiction for another, meaning patients must take methadone every day or they will begin to feel withdrawal symptoms. On the surface, this argument seems to make sense. But the critics, many of whom have no experience helping patients addicted to heroin, do not differentiate between people who are *treated with methadone and stable* and people who are *addicted to methadone*. Both groups take methadone every day, but that may be the only similarity between them. Many people confuse physical dependence with addiction. You are physically dependent on a drug if you take it every day. You can be physically dependent on high blood pressure medication, antidepressants, and methadone. Physical dependence can accompany addiction, but by itself it is not addiction.

If you are addicted to methadone, you have symptoms of addiction: You are constantly preoccupied with getting the drug; are intoxicated or euphoric; have an unstable, often negative mood; and are unable to focus on other daily activities. These symptoms are not characteristic of a patient properly treated with methadone. Many people on methadone lead incredibly stable, satisfying lives. The American Psychiatric Association has published clear diagnostic criteria for opioid use disorder (see page 60), which is understood as an addiction. A great majority of patients treated with methadone do not meet the criteria for opioid use disorder.

Decades of evidence shows that stopping medication prematurely drives relapse and death rates, and many people who stay on medication do not experience OUD symptoms. The most tragic stories are those of patients who did well on medication but stopped under outdated program rules or insurance barriers, or when prompted by their family, and then relapsed. Requiring a patient to stop taking medication for a chronic disorder based on a nonmedical argument would never be acceptable in any other field of medicine. Despite the Mental Health Parity and Addiction Equity Act passed in 2008—which is meant to ensure that people seeking mental health or substance use disorder treatment receive benefits similar to those offered for medical or surgical needs—medication barriers remain a most unfortunate reality in the treatment of opioid addiction.

Gasping for Air

Asking a heroin user to stop thinking about heroin is like asking a drowning person to stop trying to catch a breath of air. With the right medication, cravings quietly subside, and more thoughtful decisions are easier to make. People who for years could not stop thinking about drugs are once again coherent and see the need to abandon the people, places, and things associated with their drug cues. The medication gives them access to some air, enough to start thinking about how they can get to shore.

The twenty-plus-year opioid overdose epidemic—among the most deadly in US history—has continued unabated largely because of a languid, low-tech response that has failed not only our people and communities but science itself. We have at our disposal three FDA-approved, lifesaving medications for the treatment of opioid dependence, yet these medications, along with quality addiction care based on scientific advances, remain out of reach for the great majority of afflicted individuals. Most of those lucky enough to find themselves in an addiction program receive an outdated and ineffective treatment of brief detoxification followed by a nonmedical abstinence-only approach. As a result, broad swaths of the population—more than two million opioid-addicted souls eager for help—remain untreated, undertreated, or vulnerable to relapse, often with fatal consequences.

The advent of death-dealing synthetic opioids on the black market has laid waste to these vulnerable individuals much like a blazing fire burning through a dehydrated forest. For two decades, much of our nation has remained ambivalent, looking past the most effective intervention: evidence-based medical treatment. It was necessary earlier. Now, it is imperative.

This chapter's story of Eric is a common example of how someone like a college-bound football star ends up snorting heroin—and in many cases panhandling, stealing, or resorting to prostitution to pay for drugs. Eric is your neighbor, the kid in the same class as your daughter; he is your nephew or your son. Erics are everywhere. They are not depraved hedonists who lack morals. Rather, they find little or no pleasure in taking opioids, just a few hours of relief. They have taken a drug their body cannot handle. More than anyone, they want to escape their wall-less prison. But they cannot. Not on their own and not through traditional treatment methods that work for other addictions. Opioid addiction is far too cunning and baffling.

To see the present clearly, as well as learn from our mistakes, we sometimes need to look back in time. The United States has faced this and similar problems before. Allow me to walk you through two previous epidemics, to witness how they unfolded and reached closure.

CHAPTER 2

Opioid Use in America: How We Got Here

Most **people would** not use "opioids" and "American history" in the same sentence. Yet opioid use has been a part of the American fabric since colonial times, its popularity rising and waning in cycles. How this nation responded to each lingering cycle of opioid use changed over the years, alternating from offering champagne cures to imprisoning physicians and banning drugs. While some efforts may have worked to subdue a given cycle, others did more harm than good. There's a great deal we can learn from past successes and failures when responding to the nation's current public health emergency.

America's First Drug Epidemic

America's first opioid epidemic was eerily similar to today's crisis in that it began with not recreational but medicinal use. This first epidemic centered on morphine, which was first isolated from opium in 1803. In 1853, with the invention of the hypodermic syringe, morphine could be injected for fast pain relief. Injecting also produced an instant euphoria, or rush, that was not possible with other routes of administration. The syringe, a godsend to patients who required surgery or suffered serious injury, would also prove to be the method of delivery most likely to lead to addiction.

In the mid-1800s, the term *medicinal* was used quite loosely. Drug peddlers, who needed neither a degree nor expertise, marketed patent medicines that contained untold amounts of poppy-derived substances for ailments ranging from migraines to dysentery. Any quack on the street could sell them to passersby. By the time of the Civil War (1861–1865), opium and morphine lined many medicine cabinets in the form of laudanum (a common tincture of alcohol, water, and opium) or morphine powders and pills. On the battlefield, injectable morphine and morphine pills were invaluable in easing the suffering of at least some wounded soldiers. The effect of morphine's widespread distribution was apparent after the war, when thousands of soldiers found themselves addicted to the drug.

However, in the nineteenth century, women, not veterans, made up the largest number of opium and morphine addicts. Doctors regularly prescribed laudanum for menstrual cramps and migraines. At the time, addiction was recognized not as a disorder but as a moral weakness or bad habit, like gambling or swearing. No one really knew how to deal with it, yet people afflicted with opioid addiction were generally tolerated.

America's first opioid epidemic, which lasted from about 1865 to 1895, affected mostly whites, as blacks had very limited access to medical care. The drug of choice was morphine. But that soon gave way to an even stronger opioid.

Enter Heroin

Heroin, which is four times more potent than morphine when injected, first showed up in America in 1898, bottled as a cough suppressant blatantly and innocently labeled "Heroin." Some experts touted it as non-addictive (though researchers did come to the opinion that heroin *was* highly addictive and could lead to "deplorable results") and not nearly as effective a painkiller as morphine. Initially, the producers of heroin (Bayer, as in Bayer Aspirin) distributed it as a low-potency elixir, pill, pastille, or tablet to treat respiratory disorders, such as whooping cough, bronchitis, and consumption. Physicians rarely gave potent injections, and so it was not a great source of medical addiction.

But if heroin as a healing agent did not create addicts, heroin as a recreational agent did. By the start of World War I, heroin was an established street drug cheaper than opium. The Prohibition Act of 1920, which forbade the production and sale of alcohol, opened the door to even more heroin use by people looking for a substitute high.

Attempts to Stop Opioid Use and Addiction

Most drug epidemics do not completely end but subside and then linger, leaving a trail of new drugs for a new generation of people, usually teenagers and young adults looking to experiment. America's first opioid epidemic didn't really end but faded away. First, by the turn of the twentieth century, addicted Civil War veterans had either passed or were nearing the end of life—and so a generation of opioid users was dying off. Second, in 1906, the US government under President Theodore Roosevelt passed the Pure Food and Drug Act, which required that all products display a list of their ingredients as well as meet certain purity standards. At the time, the idea of giving the federal government so much power was radical. But it was the Progressive Era, and an active and vocal Pure Foods Movement begun in the 1870s had ensured that most people understood that the use of opium, morphine, and heroin could have devastating consequences. After 1906, patent medicines that listed addictive substances as ingredients were left on the shelves to collect dust. But listing an ingredient is not the same as banning it, and so those who wanted morphine still had access.

Government intervention helped limit the number of new cases of addiction, but at the time, addiction was understood far less than it is today. For the most part, attempts to help addicted individuals failed miserably. Patent medicines claiming to cure addiction contained some of the hair of the dog, as it were, including morphine and alcohol. Some were even poisonous, with such ingredients as strychnine. Withdrawal, rest in a sanatorium, fresh air, and exercise, along with champagne and port wine, were also encouraged. Those who could not afford treatment tried to go "cold turkey" at home or were sent to psychiatric asylums. Relapse was the norm, as none of the treatments worked in the long term, but many a proprietor got rich off claiming to have the cure.

Some physicians, however, latched onto yet another form of treatment that wasn't necessarily the most effective (and not always provided for the right reasons) but that they thought had potential: the narcotic clinic. In these specialized clinics, opium was prescribed to alleviate withdrawal symptoms, and morphine was given chronically to help people addicted to morphine. Doctors ran the clinics almost like the methadone programs of today. People addicted to opioids lined up two to three times a day to get a short fix. Giving addicted people their drug of choice, in the same way they took it before, might not have done much to quell the desire to keep using, but it had a stabilizing effect. These folks had access to a doctor and medical care, so the harms of using were reduced. They weren't given enough to overdose. And they were surviving. It didn't work for everyone, but at least it was a stab at a *medical* rather than a *criminal* solution.

Criminalization and antidrug campaigns were also used to curb usage, but these efforts sometimes backfired. When, in 1909, the US government tried to stop opium use by outlawing the substance, opium smoking became fashionable among the wealthy, who could afford the now higher prices. The poor and middle class turned to cheaper drugs: namely, the much harsher heroin. Amid growing concern, the government passed the Harrison Act of 1914, which in essence created a model for how *not* to treat addiction. About 5,000 doctors were imprisoned for prescribing an opioid in an effort to help a patient, regardless of whether that treatment was beneficial. Terrified, doctors either closed their narcotic clinics or secretly sold the contraband. This fostered the birth of the pill mill—a place where anyone with cash can buy a doctor-prescribed narcotic, whether medically advised or not.

The police, rather than the traditional medical board, started overseeing doctors, which created a great deal of fear within the medical profession. What stems from fear usually creates more problems, and this phenomenon had the unintended effect of hurtling the treatment of opioid addiction straight into the Dark Ages. The nation moved away from treating addiction as a medical problem to seeing it as a criminal act. Doctors and their addicted patients were prosecuted, and the whole profession of taking care of the addicted was decimated: Treating addiction with opioid medications was illegal, and if you prescribed opioids or a painkiller to patients who could not stop using, you were prosecuted if you were caught.

The last narcotic clinic closed its doors in 1921. Over the following decades, researchers explored everything from carbon dioxide therapy to LSD as ways to treat opioid addiction. It would take fifty years and another bloody war before a viable medical treatment for people addicted to opioids surfaced—or rather, resurfaced.

Opioids as Treatment

Prescribing opioids to someone with a known opioid addiction remains illegal to this day. Earlier laws guiding addiction treatment were renewed in the 1970s and most recently in 2000. There are, however, two exceptions: methadone and buprenorphine can be dispensed by a specially registered opioid treatment program, and buprenorphine can be prescribed by a medical provider with a special certification and a waiver to treat opioid addiction with an opioid without having to register as a methadone program.

The Psychedelic Sixties and Seventies: A Return to the Medical Model

The US government banned heroin in 1924, except for use in severe medical cases. But as a street drug, heroin never went away. The end of World War II and the Korean War brought about a dramatic rise in heroin use. By the 1960s, heroin use increased, in part because a large number of baby boomers were at that age when youths typically experiment with drug use. Inner-city crime, much of it drug related, was at an all-time high, and a generation of youths was dropping out and nodding off. The other, more sensitive, issue was that Vietnam War veterans were coming home with a proclivity and vulnerability for using heroin, which was readily available and widely used in the war zone by servicemen to cope with the pain and trauma of combat. Much of the nation struggled to see young soldiers coming home and injecting heroin. They had fought for the country, and their use was not a moral failing, but stress and trauma related. The government did not see these veterans as hoodlums but as heroes.

In 1969, an estimated 315,000 Americans were addicted to heroin. A short two years later, the number of addicted reached 560,000. Although these numbers pale in comparison to today's epidemic, they were staggering at the time and had nearly managed to outpace the nation's first (and much longer) opioid epidemic. Something had to be done. Smack dab in the middle of the largest crime and drug crisis since the beginning of the century, President Richard Nixon and his advisers advocated methadone treatment.

Methadone, a synthetic opioid, first came about during World War II, when the rigors of war rendered opium in short supply but the need to treat pain was only expanding. German scientists looking for a morphine substitute fabricated it from scratch. Methadone is a narcotic similar to other opioids, but it produces only minimal intoxication when taken orally and regularly. It also performs an impressive backflip: When taken daily, it reduces craving and alleviates withdrawal symptoms in OUD patients. The patient feels completely normal. If the patient is then exposed to another opioid such as heroin, they are not able to feel the high.

The Germans never used methadone as a painkiller. Their tests showed too many side effects. But postwar, a refined version of the drug made its way into the United States as a prescription painkiller. By the 1970s, because of its unique qualities, including limited euphoria and long duration of action, methadone had become a first line of treatment for heroin addiction during the nation's second opioid epidemic, which favored heroin.

The Nixon administration poured millions of dollars into addiction treatment programs. The government expanded treatment with methadone and funded research to develop alternative medical strategies, including naltrexone and later buprenorphine. This event marked the beginning of the modern, medically focused approach to treatment of opioid addiction. Prior to that, "medical" treatments of heroin addiction had been not only mostly unproven but also ineffective, dangerous, and potentially lethal.

The Birth of Methadone Maintenance Therapy

It all started with a program in New York City, which in the 1960s was the heroin capital of the United States. The idea of using methadone as a medicine to treat opioid addiction was first conceived by Dr. Vincent Dole, an endocrinologist who saw opioid addiction as a metabolic disorder of the brain that required sustained medical management to correct, though not cure, abnormalities. In other words, Dole saw addiction as a scientific problem with a scientific solution. He, along with Drs. Marie Nyswander and Mary Jeanne Kreek, both physicians working at Rockefeller University, developed and implemented methadone maintenance therapy (MMT), which involved dispensing liquid methadone to heroin-addicted individuals from specialized clinics.

Patients maintained on methadone would line up each morning in front of the clinic window, where a nurse would dispense the daily dose of methadone adjusted for each patient. For many patients, the dosage was not sedating but enough to keep cravings and withdrawal at bay. Large numbers of MMT patients went to work and led reasonably normal lives—and many of these first patients continue to do so today. MMT did not work for all, however. Some continued to use heroin or other drugs despite high doses of methadone and weekly counseling. But overall, the methadone-based treatment had the lowest failure rate of any program for treating opioid addiction: 30 to 40 percent of patients had minimal to no benefits from methadone treatment compared to 70 to 90 percent failure in other programs.

Methadone clinics, which are now known as opioid treatment programs (OTPs), had a strong initial foothold in the recovery movement. Counseling was an essential component of treatment, and many counselors were patients themselves and served as role models. Treatment was as much about the improved health, wellness, and quality of life as it was about reducing crime, demand for the drug, and overdose incidents, which were alarmingly high. In the mid-1970s, more than 650 people died every year from a heroin-related death in New York City alone. By comparison, the New York City Health Department reported a similar rate of 630 deaths in 2011, though by 2016 this figure had more than doubled.

As the reach of the methadone programs grew, the focus of treatment began to shift, from the remission of addiction and personal recovery to a reduction of harms to society (crime, costs, and safety). Disconnected from the idea of an abstinence-based recovery, MMT was a means to manage the swelling tide of heroin users from all walks of life, all across the country.

By 1984, three thousand programs were treating opioid dependence in the United States. Some programs began offering naltrexone, an opioid blocker given to patients after detoxification to prevent relapse, as an alternative to methadone. Other programs offered psychiatric, faith-based, or Twelve Step approaches, as well as long-term residential treatment in therapeutic communities such as Daytop. None of these approaches was overly successful in treating OUD except in a small group of patients.

Methadone Under Fire

Methadone clinics are still helping to save lives and reduce harm. But they are not without controversy. Methadone is a powerful medicine with side effects and a potential for harm if not used properly. Treatment with methadone also keeps patients physically dependent on opioids, meaning that they have to take the medicine every day or will suffer an unpleasant opioid withdrawal. If taken in a higher dose than prescribed, methadone can produce intoxication or even death, especially if taken in combination with other sedatives or alcohol. Because of these similarities to heroin, and a disconnection of methadone treatment from the focus on personal recovery, critics view methadone programs as "exchanging" one addiction for another—addiction to heroin for addiction to methadone.

This reaction, in fact, was nearly universal, with the notable exception of Bill Wilson, cofounder of Alcoholics Anonymous (AA), the first Twelve Step program. In a 1991 editorial entitled "Addiction as a Public Health Problem," Dr. Vincent Dole wrote the following: "[Bill Wilson] spoke to me of his deep concern for the alcoholics who are not reached by AA, and for those who enter and drop out and never return. . . . He suggested that in my future research I should look for an analogue of methadone, a medicine that would relieve the alcoholic's sometimes irresistible craving and enable him to continue his progress in AA toward social and emotional recovery, following the Twelve Steps."

Still, MMT was under fire. Negative portrayals of inner-city programs in the press further stigmatized methadone clinics. To this day, most communities are loath to permit one to operate in the area, for fear they will attract heroin dealers looking for customers like bees to honey. Strict regulations have made the clinics bureaucratic nightmares. In response to problems seen in some methadone programs that became profitable "methadone mills," the government clamped down on methadone clinics. Nowadays, multiple governmental agencies issue regulations and provide oversight. Setting up a new methadone clinic can take more than a year, and treatment is often guided by regulations more than patient needs. Being maintained on methadone still produces stigma, not only from neighbors, but from others in recovery from addiction, from families, and even from some medical professionals.

Despite these setbacks, methadone is considered the gold standard of opioid addiction treatment worldwide. Even such countries as China and Iran, initially reluctant to embrace this model of treatment, are now rapidly scaling up efforts to establish methadone clinics. Leaders are seeing the benefits to individuals and society. As part of an effort coordinated by the United Nations Office on Drugs and Crime, I am helping to train medical providers to implement methadone treatment programs in Afghanistan, one of many places where effective opioid treatment is very much needed, as approximately 5 percent of the population is using opioids. Some countries, however, most prominently Russia, remain adamantly opposed to using potentially addictive substances to treat addictions.

From Heroin to AIDS

MMT did not end the heroin epidemic—in 1986, an estimated 500,000 Americans were addicted to heroin, a number just shy of the 1971 figure—although it certainly improved a lot of lives. MMT also helped to demonstrate the utility of a medical approach. Like the earlier narcotic clinics, methadone maintenance has a strong component of harm reduction as the first step in preventing adverse health consequences. By eliminating the need for needles and transactional sex, for example, methadone maintenance protects former heroin users from the likelihood of contracting HIV/AIDS. However, it can go beyond harm reduction and allow some patients to "live self-directed lives, and strive to reach their full potential," which is the Substance Abuse and Mental Health Services Administration's definition of "recovery." But make no mistake. Addiction was still highly stigmatized as a deviant and criminal behavior and still not seen as a medical condition requiring medical attention.

The heroin epidemic, like the nation's earlier opioid epidemic, gradually faded away for three major reasons: First, many Vietnam vets gave up heroin once the trauma of the war began to subside and the triggers that encouraged drug use slowly disappeared. Veterans settled in at home with their families and at their new jobs. Second, by the mid-1980s, new drug users preferred cocaine, which ignited a new drug epidemic. And third, the AIDS epidemic was well under way, discouraging the use of disease-transmitting needles.

Lessons from the AIDS Epidemic

In 1981, AIDS was a new disease that the Centers for Disease Control and Prevention described as "a rare pneumonia contracted by young gay men." Soon afterward, intravenous heroin users and sex workers were also identified as high risk for contracting HIV. Within sixteen months of the first reported case, 40 percent of people diagnosed with AIDS were dead. While scientists struggled to find the cause and treatment, the gay community quickly mobilized, creating a movement to fund-raise for research and pressure the government to speed up the development of drugs to counteract the HIV virus, which gradually destroys the immune system of infected individuals.

Massive efforts went into training clinicians to treat viral infections in immunity-compromised patients. In 1987, with the release of the first HIV/AIDS medication, Congress provided $30 million in emergency funding to states to pay for the medications. This evolved into the AIDS Drug Assistance Program, which now exists in every US state and territory. The powerful and proactive grassroots organizations used their money and connections to ensure HIV/AIDS patients received medications at no cost. Grants were used to pay for treatment and campaigns initiated against stigma and misinformation. The AIDS epidemic went very quickly from being thought of as a stigmatized disease or a punishment for moral depravity to a disease that needed to be stopped—akin to any transmittable disease, such as tuberculosis.

As HIV/AIDS spread globally, the world, it seemed, was rooting for a cure. When medications became available, the medical community implemented them immediately on a massive scale, and the rate of deaths decreased dramatically in the United States. Most people accepted HIV/AIDS as a chronic disease that required lifelong treatment on medication, and sensationalizing the lifestyles of affected individuals gradually stopped. Moralizing, waving fingers turned into compassionate, helping hands. Even the religious right saw the urgency. HIV/AIDS had been mainstreamed, and this perspective encouraged funding and treatment. In 2016, the 21st International AIDS Conference took place, reflecting the ongoing impact of the large-scale, coordinated efforts to ensure that those with the infection continue to receive help.

HIV/AIDS hasn't gone away, but the number of lives lost to it has seen a dramatic decline. At its height in 1995, 50,000 people lost their lives to an AIDS-related illness; two years later, after the highly active antiretroviral treatment was introduced, annual deaths were down to approximately 20,000. Today, just over one million Americans are living with HIV, the number of new infections decreased by 18 percent between 2008 and 2014, and fewer than 7,000 people died in 2014 directly because of HIV.

In Europe, opioid addiction is viewed in the same way that AIDS is now seen in America: as a medical problem that requires medical attention, funding to provide free or subsidized treatment, research to improve medical treatments, and compassionate support. The United States is not quite there yet. Close to 2.5 million Americans have OUD, and about 400,000 have died from an opioid-related condition since 1999, despite the fact that there are three FDA-approved medications to treat OUD and prevent overdose deaths. Only a small percentage of individuals living with OUD receive proper treatment.

Although President Donald Trump declared the opioid epidemic a national emergency in August 2017, two months later he downgraded it to a public health emergency, which carries less weight in terms of funding. As of this writing, various commissions have outlined recommendations, and some additional money has started flowing into the system. At the same time, budget cuts have decreased funding for the Substance Abuse and Mental Health Services Administration, the nation's leading addictions agency. Furthermore, tax cuts will subject millions of people to losing health insurance coverage, including for addiction treatment. Meanwhile, the rate of overdose deaths is accelerating. More than forty-two thousand people died from opioid use in 2016, a figure that is neck and neck with deaths from the AIDS epidemic at its peak. The US moved much faster in its response to the HIV/AIDS epidemic than it has through the current opioid overdose epidemic. OUD is a different disorder, but it requires the same kind of dynamic to effect change.

The Painful Steps Leading to the Current Epidemic

The current opioid epidemic started within the medical community with good intentions—to relieve pain in patients. But a confluence of seemingly unrelated factors created a powerful, unstoppable force. It started with prominent pain doctors, who had little training in addictions, advocating that painkillers could be used safely in most patients and would not cause addiction. They pushed for primary care providers, most of whom also have little to no training in addiction, to offer opioid pain treatment to people in chronic pain—a group long believed to be underserved by the medical community. This might have worked were the prescribing done under the supervision of addiction specialists, but that is not what happened. Prior to the 1980s, opioids were primarily used in end-of-life care for patients with terminal illness. In the late 1990s, the indications for use of prescription opioids were expanded to many medical conditions: everything from wisdom teeth removal to fibromyalgia. But the evidence for their effectiveness in those new indications was minimal, and the risks underestimated.

During this same period, the medical establishment operated by a few guiding principles that were, again, not based on any systematic evidence. Medical tradition asserted that:

- Opioids used for pain are contraindicated for patients with a history of addiction, but they are generally safe for patients without such a history.
- As long as patients use opioids for pain, their addictive potential is very low (and they will not escalate doses).

- The potential for addiction is low in patients who do not have psychiatric problems.

But none of these three generalizations is true. Anyone can fall prey to addiction. Chronic treatment with opioid painkillers eventually leads to tolerance and, in most people, the dosage must be increased or the pain addressed some other way. Lastly, physicians prescribing opioids for pain grossly underestimated how many patients presenting with pain have a co-occurring psychiatric problem, where additional caution is warranted. This was compounded by an unfounded belief that medical practitioners without psychiatric training would be able to recognize people who might be at risk of addiction and not offer opioids to them. In practice, it turned out to be much more difficult. People can excel at hiding what they do not want others to know, and addiction or addictive behaviors can be difficult to spot even by the trained professional. Overall, the addictive potential of opioids used for pain was grossly underestimated. Frequently, prescribing physicians neither informed patients about the risk of addiction nor implemented plans to monitor aberrant behavior and minimize the risk.

Seemingly innocent changes in health care, meant to bring more compassionate care, silently fueled the epidemic as well. In an effort to make the patient experience more respectful and meaningful, hospitals and clinics began employing the principles of patient-centered care, which include showing respect for patients' preferences. This paved the way to patient self-report, which was ultimately seen as more valid than the objective finding of the physician. In the case of pain, the overarching belief became "pain is whatever the patient says it is." Pain assessment then became an essential part of a medical evaluation, the same way that taking body temperature, heart rate, and blood pressure are. This practice gave complaints of pain a new prominence and focus, and, with a patient-centered approach to treatment, pain relief suddenly became a primary treatment goal. There was also a cultural shift. As a whole, people were moving away from accepting pain as an inevitability of aging.

The discovery of pain necessitated the plan to relieve it: Pain-free living became the expectation.

Along with the recognition of pain, the mandate to treat it, reassurance about the safety of painkillers, and the ability of doctors to prescribe them widely (with little restriction) came efficient market forces advertising very powerful, newly formulated painkillers to doctors and patients alike, using strategies that were not only ethically questionable but also based on little scientific evidence. The fact that painkillers are highly desirable and many individuals are willing to pay a lot of money for them further drove up development, marketing, and sales of many "me-too" drugs, or drugs that duplicate the action of popular drugs already on the market. Once those market forces were unleashed, they were impossible to rein in, despite legal penalties.

Too Little, Too Late

Despite the fact that problems with prescription opioids develop in a large number of patients, known now for more than ten years, there was no change in guidelines or teaching about the use of these medications until 2016, when the CDC came out with a report that advocated for prescribing low doses for a short period of time. That is, if the opioids do not relieve pain, physicians are to stop prescribing them and look for something else. Accepting and enforcing these guidelines is another story. It is much easier to identify patients at risk, and treat them much more safely, than it is to manage those who have already developed a disorder, which then becomes chronic. As a result of these new pain treatment guidelines, fewer individuals will become addicted, but these guidelines will have little impact on people who are already addicted and might have already switched to heroin. For those who still have pain and have also developed OUD, we need to develop more promising therapeutic interventions.

What happens next is like clockwork: Once a patient is addicted to painkillers, and then finds access to painkillers restricted, it would be rare that the patient would not seek an alternative source to acquire the much-needed substance, as either heroin or pills one can get on the black market, which are often counterfeit. And most patients who use heroin will, over time, switch to more economical routes of administration, such as injecting. When high or seeking a fix, good judgment takes a backseat, and so next come risky behaviors, such as needle sharing and transactional, frequently unsafe sex. Down the road, the addicted individual seeks even cheaper and stronger opioids, such as fentanyl, and the risk of a deadly overdose escalates.

Most people who develop OUD will have a lifelong condition. Despite our having the necessary treatment to slow down the number of new cases, the overall number of people living with OUD will continue to grow, creating an increasingly large burden upon society, even though as many as 50 percent will perish after living thirty or so years with an active disorder. But if people decide to support and become vocal about a different approach to taking care of opioid-addicted individuals, we can drastically reduce all costs associated with OUD, including lives.

Asking Physicians to Turn the Tide

Physicians are expected to relieve pain. However, most are not trained, authorized, or even interested in treating addiction, because they do not consider it to be a public health issue in the same way that other chronic disorders are. Only about 4 percent of the 950,000 physicians in the United States are trained, certified, and prescribing buprenorphine, and 40 percent of US counties do not have a single buprenorphine provider. Even fewer physicians offer XR-naltrexone, another medication that can be used outside of specialty opioid treatment programs. Methadone programs number 1,400, but these are very unevenly distributed. Most are located in large cities, and half of all counties in the United States have no methadone program at all.

Much of the reluctance to treat OUD has to do with lack of training, as well as the prevailing stigma, myths, and misunderstandings about addiction. Some doctors in community health centers envision threatening or cunning heroin addicts, who haven't bathed in weeks, nodding off or disrupting the office waiting room. These providers drop the idea of offering OUD treatment altogether. Yet treating OUD is no different than treating the many other chronic disorders that doctors manage every day. Many patients have uncomplicated OUD and respond to treatment promptly and fully.

Getting certified to prescribe buprenorphine requires eight hours of training for physicians and twenty-four hours for nurse practitioners and physician assistants, and many organizations that provide training also offer ongoing mentoring to help new providers as they begin to prescribe the medication. One of such efforts is Providers' Clinical Support System (pcssnow.org), a federally funded project with a national reach. This program, which I am a part of, offers free training and support to all health-care professionals who would like to provide patients addicted to opioids with evidence-based care. In my experience of mentoring others through this program, prescribing buprenorphine to treat OUD is a relatively straightforward undertaking for most medical practitioners. After treating ten to twenty patients, most doctors get a general sense for medication effectiveness and how to minimize the risks. They begin to feel quite comfortable expanding it to many more patients. Physicians who begin working with this population find themselves pleasantly surprised at how rewarding it is. Excuses such as being too busy, not getting reimbursed, or not having a therapist on staff fall to the wayside.

France went through an epidemic of intravenous heroin use in the late 1990s. Overdoses took a dive after 20 percent of the country's physicians began prescribing buprenorphine to opioid addicts. Imagine the difference we could make in the United States if its doctors could mobilize a similar effort. Keeping addicted people at arm's length is no longer an option.

Comparing the Epidemics

So, how can we compare the first and second opioid epidemics, as well as the AIDS epidemic, with today's crisis? The first opioid epidemic was a medical epidemic. The response was at first commercial, then medical, and then criminal. Between morphine and heroin, that crisis lasted fifty years. The next big epidemic was recreational. The response was medical as well as criminal. It lasted about twenty-five years. The response to the AIDS epidemic was medical, political, and humanitarian. It lasted fifteen years before the United States was able to mount a massive and coordinated public health response and rapidly reverse its course, and for many of those years it was an unknown disease with no known treatments.

Today's epidemic is a medical epidemic. We are moving away from a criminal approach to a limited medical one, administering naloxone to reverse overdoses. But we fail the majority of people by sending them to treatment centers that do not use evidence-based treatment for opioid addiction. This opioid epidemic is nearly twenty-five years in the making and shows no signs of stopping. It has moved from opioid painkillers to heroin to fentanyl. The latest wave adds stimulants, such as methamphetamine, into the mix, which will be even harder to treat because we know little about the combination.

We've seen that epidemics don't end entirely. They fade away and linger, meaning someone always needs help. Criminalizing drug use can help to stop the flow of an illegal substance, but punishing people for having a disorder does nothing to help them or advance treatment. The advocates for AIDS treatment knew this. They pooled their resources for the higher good and made a direct impact, saving millions of lives. In that regard, OUD is similar to AIDS. It is a disease that needs treating, and we must combat stigma and ignorance until the acceptance of treatment and the number of professionals willing to engage in it will be sufficient.

Drug epidemics come and go in cycles, but the problem of addiction never really goes away: As long as there are drugs, there will be people who get addicted. But why do some people get addicted, whereas others do not? And is anyone safe from opioids?

CHAPTER 3

Opioid Use Disorder— A Disease Like Any Other?

It is Christmas Eve. Lacey and her three daughters eat dinner, finish the dishes, and tidy up before realizing that Jason is unresponsive. Jason has overdosed for the umpteenth time after downing a handful of Vicodin.

Like that of a highly decorated military hero, Jason's chest is carpeted in patches—only his are plain white and contain fentanyl. Each medicated patch releases the drug for three days, but Jason amasses the patches on his chest over several weeks, in case there is a chance he can absorb more from them. Lacey has never seen him eat a patch, although she heard at an Al-Anon meeting that it has been done.

In the early nineties, Jason had begun using opioids to help with back pain. A doctor friend prescribed some painkillers to help take the edge off. Before the opioid prescription frenzy that started in the midnineties, Jason's opioid use was manageable—even hidable. That's when he met and married Lacey. They had a good marriage, raised three smart daughters, and enjoyed a healthy community of friends. Outwardly, they were a model family, ever cheerful and happy to help anyone in need. No one knew, not even Lacey, that the last two years of their marriage would be complete and utter hell.

Twenty years prior to Jason's Christmas Eve binge, at the age of thirty, Jason suffered a snowboarding injury that left him disabled and no longer able to work. Jason became depressed and anxious. Before long, he was sitting in front of the TV 24/7, eating black market painkillers like popcorn and nodding off.

Now, on Christmas Eve, paramedics take Jason to the ER for overdose. From there, he is transferred to a hospital for detoxification, where he spends the first four days blacked out. Eight days later, Lacey comes to pick him up.

"You should be dead," the physician says to Jason as he sits glumly. "Your beautiful wife here should be planning your funeral." The doctor, who is no stranger to seeing opioid addicts, feels no need to mince words.

What Defines a Disorder?

From the outside looking in, it might seem as if addiction were a disorder of selfishness or even insanity. But if you compare addiction with other disorders, the concept is the same: Like any other medical condition, addiction has signs (drug taking, nodding off, cold sweats), symptoms (inability to stop thinking about the drug, anxiety), and a target organ (the brain). Drug use takes a direct hit against one of our most precious organs, and one that cannot be replaced. Over time, regular drug use alters brain chemistry, more dramatically in people with a genetic predisposition, creating conditions that promote more use—drugs activate parts of the brain responsible for memory and appetitive drive and suppress the part of the brain responsible for curbing urges and harmful behaviors.

Believing that addiction is a disorder rather than a voluntary choice sometimes requires a leap of faith. The families of affected individuals remain confused and angry for a long time about the inexplicable change in their loved ones' behavior, the choices they are making, and their seeming unwillingness to return to the old way of behaving. Because people using opiates can remain rational in most other areas of their lives, it seems that their behavior around drugs is knowing and deliberate. With that, most families reject the reasoning that drug use has become involuntary and compulsory. They become angry rather than compassionate, accusatory rather than supportive. They initially reject the comparison to other medical disorders as well. Only over time do they begin to accept it.

But the evidence does not lie. Brain-imaging studies that evaluated the activity of areas of the brain involved in maintaining uncontrollable drug use show changes in function as compared to otherwise healthy brains, just as imaging studies show decreased function in the areas of the heart muscle where blood flow is blocked. In parallel, studies show reversal of these "abnormal" changes in the brains of patients who are able to remain drug free for more than six months as compared with the brains of patients with only days of abstinence. Other studies show that medications effective in treating drug addiction not only block specific receptor sites but also reverse deficits in the functioning of key brain centers. While it is difficult to identify brain areas that are only responsible for addictive behaviors, the fact that there is a predictable brain activity with the emergence and resolution of the disorder supports the fact that at the core of addiction is a disordered brain. It functions differently than the brain of an average person without the disorder.

The Best Way to Treat a Disorder

Viewing addiction as a chronic disorder not only helps dispel stigma but aids in understanding and treating the disorder. If addiction is proven to be a chronic brain disorder, our intervention should mirror the medical model for management of other chronic disorders, which allows for ongoing medical attention with a focus on long-term management, education, and support—the same model we use to treat hypertension and diabetes, for example.

Diabetics live with an impaired pancreas (the target organ) that is unable to fully control insulin levels. No matter how much diabetics try, they cannot fundamentally change how their pancreas works. And so, because we know diabetes is a chronic but treatable disease, we offer diabetics medication in the form of insulin, along with education about the best possible diet. If diabetics cannot control their craving for sugar, we adjust their insulin dosage until it stabilizes blood sugar levels. We don't give up on these patients or send them to a residential program away from their home to give them a controlled diet and correct blood sugar levels. We intervene with evidence-based treatments before the onset of the possible consequences of the disease, including kidney failure, amputation, and blindness. And we keep treating diabetics for the rest of their lives, making sure they continue taking the medicine correctly and safely but also educating and supporting them to become personally responsible for the management of their disease.

You're probably thinking that this explanation is all good and well, but none of it gets to the heart of the behavioral aspect of drug taking. Why, for instance, do people take drugs to begin with? Nor does it address why almost everyone uses substances recreationally at some point in their lives but only some become addicted, or why a once reliable person starts betraying loved ones for the sake of getting a fix. And why do addicted people, in particular, continue using despite some fairly severe negative consequences—such as getting fired or losing a toddler to child protective services? How is it possible that someone who willingly and habitually takes drugs, isolates, and not only neglects responsibilities but steals and lies in order to get high has a disorder? Lastly, why do nearly 25 percent of people using heroin develop OUD, when only 8 to 10 percent of alcohol drinkers develop alcohol use disorder?

The Power of Memory

The short answer to why people start drinking or taking other mood-altering drugs is simple: to feel *good* or feel *better*. Some do it to bring on an intense pleasure that is not otherwise available; others, to cope with daily stress, financial problems, the memory of traumatic experiences, or symptoms of a psychiatric disorder. Conversely, some, by the nature of their brains, cannot enjoy the positive effects of a given drug because the drug's adverse effects are stronger. For example, groups of people living in China and Japan have a genetic mutation that causes them to have a very unpleasant reaction to alcohol. These people find little or no pleasure in drinking. As a result, very few of them become heavy drinkers or alcoholics.

Mood-altering drugs make most us feel good or better because they make a beeline for the "pleasure center" of the brain. Once there, they mimic the effects of natural brain chemicals to produce a sense of well-being and euphoria. The pleasure center is an ancient and forceful presence. It functions by rewarding us for behaviors essential for our survival as a species. The brain releases these same "feel-good" chemicals when we eat, socialize, have sex, or exercise. They're the brain's way of encouraging us to keep doing these life-promoting activities. The feel-good chemicals stimulate the brain centers so we remember the experience and how good it made us feel, as well as the environment where these important experiences took place. All of this is to make sure we will do it again.

With each such experience, the brain changes a bit, making it easier for us to want to repeat the experience. The desire or craving that precedes the activity is there to influence our choices. Addictive drugs, however, flood the brain with chemicals that act like impostors, taking hostage of functions that exist to ensure survival. We feel good and cannot differentiate whether this feeling plays any important role in survival. We just want to repeat the experience, which can be likened, at first, to the heady feeling of falling in love, an overpowering sensation that is often stronger than our ability to reason. If we get in the habit of turning to drugs regularly to feel good or better, we find that the drugs start to lose some of their wondrous and giddy effects. All potentially addictive drugs, whether made in a lab or found in nature, eventually stop working as well when overconsumed. More and more, positive effects are replaced with negative ones. This change in drug effects over time happens faster in some people than in others.

The Importance of Tolerance and Physical Dependence

The brain does much more than promote our desires to have a good time. It preserves important functions, such as breathing and alertness. It is about survival and will adapt to preserve its most essential functions if necessary. When overwhelmed by repeated and massive amounts of drugs, your brain adapts by going into protective mode. It shuts down neurochemical receptor sites to prevent an overflow of drugs from interfering with essential brain functions. To keep you alive, your brain has *changed its function and structure*. Two of the most clinically visible brain changes are tolerance and physical dependence.

Tolerance

Tolerance is a key term in addiction medicine. It is used to describe a threshold, or how much of a drug you must consume to get the desired effect. With continued use, the threshold rises. As it rises, you need to take more drugs. For example, if you increase the number of pills consumed from, say, one to two and then six but continue to feel the same way you did when taking one, you have increased your tolerance. Your brain function has changed in an effort to prevent overdose. You now need six pills to feel the same way you did when you were taking only one pill. Although it may sound counterintuitive, tolerance is the brain's way of protecting the body against overdose. It is a defense mechanism.

The more powerful and faster the effects of the opioid, the faster tolerance develops, and the sooner you must escalate the daily dose. This is an experience known well to all drug users, whether using marijuana or painkillers.

Physical dependence

Physical dependence is another sign that the brain has adapted to the constant presence of opioids. When you are physically dependent on a drug, the brain expects the daily presence of the drug, whether prescription painkillers or heroin, to stay "in balance." Physical dependence is not addiction (although it can be a symptom of addiction), which involves another set of changes in the brain center. The opioids block the release of noradrenaline, a brain chemical that mobilizes the body in dangerous or stressful situations for the "fight or flight" response. In response, the brain exposed to opioids produces more noradrenaline, but the constant flow of opioids keeps this extra noradrenaline in check. In this way, the brain remains "in balance" as long as opioids are regularly flowing into the body from the outside.

If you are physically dependent and stop taking opioids, your system quickly goes off-balance, and you start feeling symptoms of withdrawal—aches, pains, nausea, diarrhea, insomnia, hyperactivity, and anxiety. This is a result of an overactive noradrenaline system, whose effects are no longer suppressed by opioids. In some sense, symptoms of withdrawal serve a purpose. Without opioids, your digestive, cardiovascular, and nervous systems (also adapted by and now dependent on drug use) are stressed, and your brain is doing what it can to encourage you to take more opioids so your body can preserve "normal" function. You experience this encouragement as craving. Your brain is now focused entirely on self-preservation, and all other functions go by the wayside.

Some drugs affect you more severely than others, depending on their type, dose, and the speed with which the drug reaches your brain, but all addictive substances, even alcohol, marijuana, caffeine, and nicotine, are capable of altering your brain and producing withdrawal symptoms. Depending on the severity of the withdrawal symptoms, stopping can be easier said than done.

At this point, the only thing you can do is abstain and give your brain time to heal so that it starts opening up receptor sites and producing feel-good chemicals on its own again. But with opioids, the cravings are so pronounced, and withdrawal so miserable, that abstinence seems unfathomable. And so, as much as you might want to escape your addiction, you are compelled to seek an ever-higher dose to try to feel normal. Feeling good is a thing of the past.

It's All in Your Head

Addiction is not as simple as drinking or using too much. If addiction were as simple as overconsumption, college students who binge drink would all be chronic alcoholics. But they aren't. Many of them lose interest after graduating, as their attention turns to a new chapter in their lives. Addiction also involves the mind. We become addicted by enjoying the experience. We stay addicted because our brains are capable of remembering those experiences, and we desire to repeat them. Powerful memories never go away. To stop using, our only choice is to develop new, more meaningful memories. Binge-drinking college students, for instance, might enjoy waking up without a hangover and dressing up for work better than they did getting sickeningly intoxicated, and so create new memories that gradually become more influential than previous ones.

Football as a Metaphor

Aaron Hernandez, the former New England Patriot football tight end who was convicted of murder and later committed suicide in his prison cell at the age of twenty-seven, was posthumously found to have chronic traumatic encephalopathy (CTE), a degenerative brain disease caused by repeated blows to the head. CTE is not uncommon among professional athletes who have suffered multiple concussions throughout their career. The brain disease can lead to aggressive and impulsive behavior as well as suicide. There is no test for CTE, although there are some signs and symptoms. Only an autopsy of the brain can confirm that the disease is present. Aaron's CTE was severe. Doctors compared it to the progressive CTE of NFL football players who were more than thirty years his senior. So, why didn't Aaron stop playing football when he felt himself changing?

Let's rewind a little further. First, Aaron chose to play football. Probably, like most professional athletes, he loved the sport as a kid and was good at it. So, he kept playing. As a professional, he made good money and felt elevated by the cheers of a stadium full of fans for doing what he loved—in other words, his behavior was repeatedly rewarded. He would suffer a concussion or an injury but would recover and continue to play. In other words, the adverse consequences didn't stop him because the reward was stronger. Aaron's personality started to change, the result of changes to the structure and function of his brain from years of being hit in the head during practices and games, causing him to lose control over some of his behaviors. Only after being thrown in prison for murder did Aaron stop playing football. And it wasn't by choice.

In Aaron's case, football was the drug; head trauma, the needle; and CTE, the resulting brain disorder. The injuries inherent in the game had an effect on Aaron's brain that gave him a disorder. It is true that if Aaron had chosen not to play sports, none of this would have happened. But playing football made him feel good, so he kept repeating the experience. An unfortunate combination of external events and his inability to recognize what was happening to him and stop before it was too late were what led to his demise and death.

How addiction develops is in many ways similar. As with CTE, there is no test for addiction; at first the opioid user is rewarded for repeating the experience; adverse consequences are often not enough to stop the desire to repeat the experience; and the structure of the brain changes so that the user loses the ability to stop at will, regardless of the consequences.

Opioid Use Disorder

We know far more about addiction now than we did a hundred years ago, when snake-oil cures were the rage. Guidelines for how to best understand and diagnose addiction continue to change and improve with research.

Current diagnostic criteria, established by the American Psychiatric Association, call addiction a substance use disorder (SUD). The association also calls out SUDs by the drug of choice: alcohol, cocaine, cannabis, tobacco, and opioids (opioid use disorder, or OUD). Before any individual develops SUD, they are using the substance without the signs or symptoms of addiction, sometimes for a long time, even months or years. SUD rarely develops after only a few episodes of use. More often, it develops in a step-wise progression, moving from mild to moderate and finally severe.

Determining whether someone uses opioids recreationally or has a full-blown addiction is not always easy, even for addiction experts following clear-cut guidelines. It is not as if we can draw a line in the sand and delineate that when it is crossed, addiction is present. OUD and other drug addictions follow a progression marked by twists and turns. The continuum jumps back and forth and can change month to month. To date, there is no physical test to determine whether addiction is present (although there are many physical consequences). We gather information from a clinical interview and the patient's report. We diagnose OUD and other SUDs by a set of behaviors—behaviors indicative of someone whose brain functioning has changed and who has lost the ability to control their substance use. The more consistent the presence of behaviors, and the more numerous, the more serious the disorder.

Most diagnostic standards emphasize four core components of addiction:

1. Preoccupation with the drug and strong urges to use with the loss in the ability to control the amount and duration of use
2. Escalation of drug use at the expense of other, personally and societally beneficial activities with resulting impairment of functioning
3. Continuing drug use despite significant negative consequences
4. Physical changes occurring as a result of drug use such as tolerance and physical dependence with symptoms of withdrawal

The *DSM-5* lists eleven symptoms: two to three symptoms during the prior twelve months are considered to have a mild use disorder; four to five symptoms over the same period is considered moderate use disorder; six or more symptoms equals severe. OUD may also be complicated by the presence of other psychiatric disorders, medical issues, and by many social problems. How we address each stage of OUD varies. We can work to prevent a mild opioid use disorder, for instance, by identifying individuals at risk and implementing psychoeducational interventions or initiating therapy that focuses on coping strategies. Initiating treatment early on in a disorder's progression ensures the best outcomes, prevents progression to more severe forms, and minimizes risks of serious consequences, such as infection, liver disease, overdoses, psychiatric complications, and personal losses.

Nicole's Story

It is Nicole's twenty-fifth birthday. She spends the day moving into a new apartment with Jake, her boyfriend of seven years. Nicole has been sober for about five years, minus an occasional lapse or two. She went through multiple detoxes and treatment programs, two of them residential, to finally reach the point where she is comfortable in her own skin. Although she has a drink on occasion, she is abstinent from opioids.

Jake is just out of a sober house. He has been gone for nearly a year, including the time he spent in residential treatment. After being sober for three years with Nicole, Jake relapsed to painkillers and heroin for a punishing year. Watching him deteriorate was prevention enough for Nicole, who stayed clean. Now, they are going to try to live as a couple again.

After a long day of unloading and unpacking, they go to bed. Nicole senses something is off. Jake, she can tell, is high. Too tired to fight about it, Nicole falls asleep. In the morning, Jake is not breathing. She shakes him and tries to do CPR, but she cannot move his jaw.

The paramedics arrive and get Jake's heart beating again. At the hospital, the intensive care physician tells Nicole that Jake went into cardiac arrest after taking cocaine and two bags of heroin. Before treatment, he was accustomed to taking much more. Because he had detoxed and no longer had any tolerance for the drugs, they were a complete assault on his system.

Jake is put on life support. Five days later, Nicole and Jake's family make the grueling decision to end support. Having gone so long without oxygen, Jake's body cannot be fixed.

Nicole holds it together until the funeral, but afterward turns to her old friends heroin and cocaine for comfort. Before long, she is consuming fifteen to twenty bags of heroin a day topped with a gram of cocaine. She loses thirty pounds in four months; the source of her weight loss is part grief and part drugs.

One day four months later, Nicole wakes to find her legs grossly swollen. She has no clue what is happening, and her mom shuttles her to the ER. The sonogram does not lie. Nicole is six months pregnant, carrying a healthy, three-pound fetus. Not having felt one symptom, and having lost rather than gained weight, Nicole is in shock.

Nicole has never liked using, but stopping on her own is not an option. The moment she tried cocaine at age sixteen, she was hooked and snorted at least a few lines every day. At seventeen, she tried OxyContin, and like a fickle lover, immediately dropped coke for the painkillers and used daily. By the time she was eighteen, she turned to heroin.

Nicole has never had a good day while using. She remembers only bad days. And now, again, she wakes up every morning thinking only about her next fix.

A Chronic Condition with Many Unknowns

For practical purposes, OUD can be defined as a disorder that follows a chronic course. If you have OUD, even if you undergo treatment and abstain, the risk of relapse persists. The more and longer you used, the more healing your brain must undergo. Cravings for the drug do not suddenly subside in the absence of opioids. It can take months or years—usually said to be at least five years—before you stop thinking about the drug completely. However, I see recovery as more of a continuum. Without medical support, each year of abstinence reduces the risk of relapse, yet the risk still exists. There is no way of knowing whether relapse is imminent. I tend to advise my patients that the best way to live with this unknown is to accept OUD as a chronic condition, just as you would accept diabetes.

OUD cannot be cured, but if you have it, you can return to living a "normal" life. Sustained recovery can and does happen, regardless of how many overdoses or relapses you have undergone. It is possible, even, to find a life in recovery far better than the one prior to opioid use. The key is intervention. Long-term treatment with medication, preferably in combination with psychological treatment, is without a doubt the most effective treatment available for OUD. Additional interventions, such as participation in self-help groups, is desirable and can be extremely helpful, but it cannot be suggested in lieu of medical treatment. Some people achieve and maintain long-term recovery without medication, but at this point we have no way of determining who they are. Medication-based treatment, on the other hand, is a proven approach that works for most people, which is why we should offer it as a first line of treatment to anyone in need of help.

Who Is a Candidate for Developing Addiction and OUD?

The first use of drugs is almost always a choice: the teenager who wants to fit in and takes his first sip of beer or hit of marijuana, the mom who starts drinking wine every evening after all the kids have moved out of the house, and patients taking two Percocet as needed for postsurgical pain. For a majority of people, that choice turns out to be harmless. They manage to drink socially or smoke a joint on occasion without any consequence. They take their opioids as prescribed and never contemplate going to the pharmacy for a refill. Use of alcohol or other drugs might fluctuate during periods of their life, but they have no trouble setting their drug of choice aside when responsibility calls.

Once the choice is made to use or drink, it's a little like playing Russian roulette. No one knows with 100 percent certainty whose use will become chronic and whether one drug will have more influence than another in establishing addiction. For one person it is wine. For another it is opioids. We have some indicators of who is likely to become addicted, and they are based on two separate influences: genetics and environment.

But there is no test. If you come from a family with a history of addiction, you are a candidate. If no one in your family has suffered from addiction, you are less of a candidate, although still at risk. If you lose your job, go through a divorce, or suffer a different traumatic event, you can activate dormant addiction genes, start using the substance in response to certain internal and external triggers, and start the addiction process. Likewise, if you grow up surrounded by drug use, understanding it as a normal part of life, you might use to excess and alter your brain chemistry enough to cross the line into addiction, even though you do not have many of the genes that facilitate it.

Myths About the Nature of OUD

The following statements are myths yet still widely believed:

- OUD is an acute problem that can be successfully cured over a short term (weeks to months); it is not a lifelong condition.

- Opioid withdrawal is physical but relapse is mental; relapse is a choice.

- When people are physically dependent, they are addicted, but once the physical dependency is removed, controlling use is easy.

- Most people taking opioid pills recreationally will not get addicted; pills are much safer than heroin; pills are less addictive; people cannot overdose on pills; people can only overdose if they inject.

- Children born to mothers who are taking prescribed opioids, whether for treatment of pain or OUD, will be born addicted.

- Addiction is not a disease of the brain; it is a learned behavior under full voluntary control.

- Addicted individuals have no control over their behavior.

Screening for OUD

If we cannot identify those at risk, how can we help them before it is too late? The gap between suspecting or knowing whether someone has a problem with opioids and getting them to either reduce use or enter evidence-based treatment is frustratingly wide. Frustrating because we have the effective tools necessary to narrow the gap, yet we are slow to implement them. Thousands of people are falling through the cracks. Screening and brief intervention with referral to treatment (SBIRT), a movement currently under way to close the gap, shows promise.

With SBIRT, health-care professionals can help the individuals who come to them—often in a medical clinic, pain clinic, or hospital emergency room—where they are usually being treated for other conditions. For example, although there is no test to determine whether someone has OUD—or would have it if they started taking opioids—we can screen for it and other addictions. SBIRT is kind of like Addiction 101. It's a tool any health-care professional in any setting can employ to try to catch problematic behavior early, before it becomes a major problem, and motivate the individual to change. The three-tiered model calls for an assessment using standardized screening tools. If problematic use is suspected, the provider talks about it with the patient, using a somewhat standardized script known to motivate. If the disorder is diagnosed, the doctor refers the patient to treatment or implements treatment in the current setting.

SBIRT is known to reduce use and save money. When SBIRT-trained medical professionals employ the method consistently with people who use alcohol, it has been shown to limit a full-blown progression to alcohol use disorder. Many people do not know, for instance, that having three drinks a day is considered problematic. Once they have the conversation, it is as if a lightbulb goes on, and many agree to start drinking less. Although SBIRT has not shown the same results with OUD, this could change as more professionals use SBIRT and as the help for and conversation about OUD becomes more acceptable, compassionate, and mainstream. Stigma is one of the biggest reasons why addiction is still a taboo subject: Patients don't mention it to doctors or seek help, and doctors are not asking about it. Talking about addiction is one of the best ways to reduce that stigma.

Once trained, *any* health-care professional can implement SBIRT in *any* setting, expanding outreach well beyond the grapevine, which is what many family members go through to find treatment for a loved one they believe is addicted. Early identification of problematic substance use in the medical setting is an opportunity to promptly intervene and prevent the progression of the disorder to the stage when consequences are more severe and treatment may be more difficult.

But like any tool, SBIRT is only as good as its implementation. Getting some health-care professionals and the institutions they work for to accept SBIRT has been slow. It can be difficult to change the behavior of career health-care providers who have been at it for more years than not, and so the current strategy is to target students in training. Another issue involves medical records and confidentiality. Hospitals, ever cautious about being sued, are leery of documenting drug use, lest records get subpoenaed, for instance, and inadvertently condemn the patient who is just being honest when they reveal they occasionally use cocaine and alcohol.

Because of problems with stigma and the need to protect patient confidentiality in addiction treatment programs (to decrease barriers to entering treatment), it was necessary in the past to completely separate medical and addiction records. Now that we are working harder toward integrating addiction treatment into mainstream medical care, the law that has protected patients stands in the way of helping them. Doctors barred from accessing important medical histories cannot act on them.

The benefits of SBIRT, however, outweigh the legal risks. At Columbia University, we have a program where we train medical students in SBIRT. We see firsthand how students' attitudes toward patients with SUD change. When these students become doctors, their heightened awareness and openness will make them better able to detect the disorder in patients early on. Hopefully, as doctors, they will be open to treating addicted individuals. A lot of these programs exist for medical residents, nursing residents, and nurses, in settings ranging from clinics and hospitals to public health offices, social worker services, and school services.

Harm Reduction

For those deeply mired in the world of addiction, the conversation begins not with prevention or treatment options but the delivery of free condoms, clean needles, and instructions for how to use drugs safely. This is harm reduction, or using known ways to reduce some of the risk associated with drug use. Intervening on those who suffer from severe OUD and either see no way out or have no desire to quit drugs requires a different, more subtle and basic approach. We attempt to reduce harm by protecting people who use drugs from unsafe sex and soiled needles, and thus infectious diseases, such as HIV and hepatitis C. Some harm reduction centers will test heroin brought in by clients to make sure it does not contain deadly fentanyl, offer to exchange clean syringes for dirty ones, dispense disinfectant, provide a safe space for injecting heroin, and even give naloxone to reverse an overdose if necessary. Outreach workers refer people who use drugs to places where they can find free food, clothing, and shelter.

As outreach workers develop an informal relationship built on trust, they gently try to coax users into getting help. They lend an ear, have accepting and nonjudgmental conversations, and share information about access to social or public health services. Although outreach and harm reduction might resemble a propaganda effort, they are really more altruistic—public services built on compassion and the desire to save lives and reduce the amount of heartache OUD can manifest. No one is forced into treatment. No one is arrested for being in possession of illegal substances. Survival and the preservation of human dignity outweigh all else.

Outreach workers are trained to replace social exclusion with acceptance, and as the addicted individuals open up to the positive experiences they have with an outreach worker, they open up to the idea of treatment and recovery. Even something as simple as a syringe access program, available in some states, is effective. By simply interacting with outreach workers, users are five times more likely to enter treatment.

PART 2

The Science, Practice, and Challenge of Treating OUD

CHAPTER 4

Embracing the New Medical Approach to Treating OUD

It is ten below zero in what seems like the middle of nowhere in Pennsylvania. The sun is as bright as the air is crisp. Michael is outside wearing only his lacrosse pinny and a pair of shorts.

"What are you doing out there?" a voice shouts from the doorway.

"I'm okay," Michael assures his counselor. "I can't remember the last time I felt cold, that's all."

Michael is in his third week of a twenty-eight-day stay at a residential treatment center. At twenty-three, he is already a hard-core opioid user. Completely drug- and alcohol-free for the first time since the eighth grade, Michael is testing the waters. Feeling cold, he decides, is nothing to complain about. It is exhilarating.

Michael first approached drug use like many adolescents do. At twelve or thirteen, he tried beer and vodka and then progressed to pot. He was the first of his high school friends to try ecstasy and cocaine. He liked being the first. It meant he was good at what he did.

An honor student and athlete, playing on his high school hockey and lacrosse teams, Michael, despite his love of drugs, did not suffer any seriously negative consequences. He came close—like the time when he and his friends were pulled over by police—but he talked his way out of any potential trouble and glided through high school unscathed. By age nineteen, he was already bored with the bar scene in his hometown. He was ready to start college, where he had made the hockey and lacrosse teams.

In the spring of his freshman year, the college notified Michael that he was being kicked out for failing or dropping out of four classes, but he convinced the school he would turn his grades around. He returned in his sophomore year and picked up club sports as his poor grades made him ineligible for the college teams. When he injured his foot playing the precarious position of goalie for his lacrosse team, the doctor prescribed Oxy-Contin, which Michael dutifully took. His next thought was that nothing should feel this good—and that nothing that feels this good should be in the possession of a twenty-year-old.

Before injuring his foot, Michael had never thought about opioids. He was so naive about the drug that the first time he went through withdrawal, he thought he had the flu. But he quickly became intimately familiar with what opioids can do.

Michael often quipped that his drinking and other drug use left him with a blood alcohol level higher than his GPA. He was kicked out of college before the end of the first semester of his sophomore year. Depressed and anxious, Michael woke up to find himself on the ledge outside his apartment building, between the seventh and eighth floors, with an empty bottle of Jameson in hand. (How he managed to stay atop is a mystery. He remembers nothing of his intentions. He only knows he is grateful he did not roll over in his sleep.)

Michael returned to his parents' home in New York. At six foot two, he weighed a mere 143 pounds. His Facebook friends posted photos of travel and good times, while he isolated in his room and took drugs. Months after first trying opioids, Michael now needed to crush and snort three Oxys before he could even get out of bed. His first thoughts were not *What classes do I have today and who will I meet up with?* but *Who am I going to rip off and how am I going to get my fix?*

Raised in a loving family with solid values, Michael knew that what he thought and did was against everything he was taught and held dear. He started to believe he was some kind of monster and refused to look in the mirror for a solid two years. He was loath to see who he had become. Suicidal thoughts filled his head: He would keep using for as long as he could and then jump in front of a train. (Now, when he recalls this, it is with disbelief.)

Moody and argumentative, he ruined every holiday. When confronted by family about his use, he became violent—throwing objects or yelling. His parents caught him stealing money from them on more than one occasion. The last straw was when he snatched his aunt's painkillers, given to her postsurgery, during a family weekend at a beach house. A few months later, his family intervened, and Michael was ready—more than eager—to get help.

When Michael entered the residential facility, his physician asked whether he wanted to try buprenorphine. But Michael was done with any drug containing opioids. He was done with dark thoughts. He was done with living a lie and hurting the people he loved. He went through detox and started extended-release naltrexone. And then he went outside in the cold to feel what it meant to be human again.

When Patients Begin to Blossom

There is something inherently rewarding about treating opioid users. Within two to three weeks, they undergo a profound change. They look and feel much better. Everyone around them notices that they are getting well. Helping patients addicted to cocaine or alcohol is also gratifying but different. They experience a lot of ups and downs in early recovery. People coming off opioids, however, quickly start to blossom.

We might attribute the stark difference that takes place in heroin users, in particular, to the fact that most come into treatment looking and feeling emaciated, depressed, and resigned. Most also bear a heavy load of shame. They've been through a lot to survive, often on the streets, doing things that defy even their strongest values. Sometimes for years or decades. But it does not matter how much time they have spent wasting away. In just a short time, their senses begin to wake up, and they start noticing and enjoying the little things, as well as some major physical changes. They regain their appetites, bowel functions, and libidos. Women start menstruating again. Mood quickly improves, and they want to go back to interests they abandoned as the addiction took over. They start feeling human again.

With this usually comes a backlog of emotions. Opioids level all emotions, good and bad. Most opioid users in treatment are surprised by the swelling of foreign sensations within—they feel happy, sad, excited, motivated. Sometimes all at the same time. Being witness to this is an honor in some way. It is like watching a child laugh, or just start to walk, for the first time. Then, some of them suddenly remember why they started taking opioids in the first place: social anxiety, depression, rape, no job. This proves overwhelming and produces a mounting urge to use. For some, these feelings are a formative experience. They use their feelings to become wiser, more insightful and more mature. This growth does not happen overnight. Over time, with the help of counseling and behavioral treatments, life starts to look better.

Despite the profound changes that take place early on, relapse is extremely common for people with OUD. We know that relapse is also highly dangerous for those who have detoxified. Their bodies can no longer tolerate amounts previously consumed, and they have easy access to a marketplace full of potent fixes. And so, as you know by now, I am convinced that stabilizing the OUD patient using medication is paramount at this stage, because it helps to prevent relapse, which saves lives and gives people a chance to work on recovery without the constant distraction of cravings.

But stabilization is just the beginning. A major shift has been taking place in treatment circles that embraces the medical model for treating OUD in the long term, which for some people can mean lifelong use of methadone, buprenorphine, or naltrexone.

The Major Shift in How We Treat Opioid Dependence

Over the past century, health-care professionals like myself have learned a lot about what does not work when it comes to treating OUD. Effort went into testing various ways to detoxify opioid users comfortably. We tried short detoxes and long detoxes, and we tried all sorts of remedies, many of them quite dangerous. We gave patients methadone or buprenorphine or clonidine to help wean them off opioids and then gradually tapered them off these drugs (methadone and buprenorphine were used for detoxification before they were thought of as primarily maintenance agents). Over and over again, the evidence showed that it does not really matter how effective the detoxification process is or how smoothly it goes. After we detoxified patients, most relapsed—many of them right after the detox was over. Not only did we not help patients, we heightened their chances of having a deadly overdose, as detoxification took away their tolerance for the drug.

Now we know much better: If we start patients on a medication, such as methadone or buprenorphine, with the intent to keep them on it indefinitely, most patients have a fighting chance. If patients want to change medication or modify dosages, we review their progress and consider working their goals into a treatment plan. If patients want to be fully detoxed, we detox them and then prescribe naltrexone, which is not an opioid agonist. If patients want to stop using medications, we talk about how stable their recovery is, begin to taper the medication, and carefully monitor them. If patients decide to stop their medication themselves, more likely than not they relapse.

Study after study shows medication to be the most effective way to treat OUD. But the shift to using the medical model has been so painfully slow that thousands of people die every year because so few treatment centers offer evidence-based treatment. Equally disturbing is when clinics offer medication but require that patients taper off it on a certain timeline.

Resistance to Change

Resistance to the medical model approach to treating OUD comes from two camps: patients (and sometimes their family members), and treatment providers. Rather than being happy that a medication can keep them alive and well, many patients and their loved ones reject the idea of medication as a necessary evil. Some want nothing more than to leave it behind them as soon as possible. This kind of thinking stems from a deep disappointment and difficulty accepting the loss of health. I have never met a patient who wants to be told they have a chronic disorder that requires lifelong treatment with medication, even if the medication is highly effective. This happens in traditional treatment centers as well: No one wants to hear that they have to abstain from all mood-altering drugs and attend Twelve Step meetings for the rest of their life. The idea of having a chronic condition is a hard pill to swallow. Psychiatrists know it well. It takes many years for people with bipolar disorder, for instance, to accept that they have a chronic illness and need to be on medication for the rest of their lives. Those who do not accept their illness spend their days wrecked by it.

Medication is a gift, a fruit of modern science that not only extends but remarkably improves the lives of people afflicted with OUD, a devastating disorder. If we are to overcome the opioid epidemic, every professional who engages with a person who uses opioids must embrace the individual, the evidence, and the condition for what it is: a lifelong, incurable disorder that can be managed successfully with medication.

The Evidence Is Overwhelming

Preventing relapse is a treatment priority for OUD patients. Intense cravings for opioids may last for months after stopping use, and can be powerful enough to cause a relapse. Detoxed people who take more drugs than their bodies can handle can easily overdose. Relapse prevention is synonymous with overdose prevention, with preventing death.

To win the battle, we must fight fire with fire. Anyone who offers opioid addiction treatment must let go of fanciful notions of a medication-free recovery for every patient. It occasionally happens, yes, but the evidence and the statistics do not lie. The only evidence-based method currently available to help prevent relapse to opioids is a medical model that includes long-term medication as the most essential intervention. *The evidence is overwhelming and cannot be ignored.* Centers that do not use medication to treat OUD are no match for today's opioids. Continuing to tout other treatments as effective against OUD is akin to giving patients a death sentence, and has led to lawsuits for more than one treatment center that claimed to offer effective treatment but did not follow evidence-based guidelines.

To some addiction counselors in practice today, using the medical model to treat OUD may sound heretical. But I am not some rogue advocate of this approach. All published treatment guidelines from all the major addiction groups call for using treatment that includes medication, sometimes referred to as medication-assisted treatment, or MAT, to treat opioid addiction. These groups include the US surgeon general, American Society of Addiction Medicine, Centers for Disease Control and Prevention, US Department of Veterans Affairs, and the World Health Organization, as well as a number of guidelines prepared by professional organizations in other countries. All the research literature points to what I am saying. This is nothing new. Yet government funds and insurance, including Medicaid, continue to cover the cost of traditional programs, further perpetuating the problem.

The medical model approach speaks to the current public health crisis, which is a crisis of the treatment gap and opioid overdoses. Initially, one treatment should fit the majority of patients: Stabilize patients using medication, provide support for patients to adhere to the medication, manage coexisting medical and mental health issues, and help patients develop new skills. This approach stalls the addiction and saves lives. Once a patient is stabilized and in the system of care, then we have the luxury of customizing our treatment approach.

Traditional Treatment

Twelve Step–based therapies and meetings are a meaningful path to recovery for many people, who learn to let go of resentments and behaviors that keep them using. Twelve Step meetings, such as Narcotics Anonymous, offer an accepting and supportive community, and people learn they are not alone in their disorder. Those in recovery are fortunate to have Twelve Step meetings and other supports. But for OUD, some flexibility is in order. The traditional nonmedical model of psychosocial treatment involving withdrawal management (detoxification) followed by treatment without medications should not be used as a first-line approach as it has a very high failure rate—on average, greater than 90 percent within the first three months. And detoxification without medication to prevent relapse increases the risk for overdose due to the loss of tolerance for the drug.

When combined with medication, traditional treatment approaches work for OUD. As patients engage with treatment and follow the program, their thoughts move away from craving and using. Some traditional programs, such as the Hazelden Betty Ford Foundation, have adapted their policies to combat today's formidable opioids by offering medication to their patients with OUD. Some programs have even changed their definition of sobriety to accommodate patients who are abstinent with the help of medication. But only a handful of traditional addiction treatment centers has the medical staff or funds required to administer medications, and some advocate for a short course of medication treatment before the "real" sobriety can set in. Many centers that would agree to offer medications are unable to. Or they face resistance from staff or even alumni and donors.

In the midst of the nation's worst drug crisis ever, we cannot wait for the costly and time-consuming change in attitudes and methods in treatment centers across America. We cannot wait to train a new generation of treatment providers. We are obliged, instead, to turn to other opportunities to effectively treat opioid users who want help now—namely, an existing and already highly organized system that regularly employs the medical model for chronic disorders.

A Call to Medical Professionals

Medical professionals in health-care settings can fill in the huge gap in evidence-based treatment services that exists today. Opioid users should be able to walk into their local clinic, request help for OUD, receive an assessment and medical checkup, have a conversation about treatment options, and, if the patient agrees and the doctor finds it appropriate, receive a prescription for buprenorphine on the spot. The same could happen every time an opioid user overdoses and lands in a medical setting. At a follow-up appointment, the physician and patient can discuss next options, which are much easier to plan and execute when the patient's mind is clear, or at least not filled with intense urges to use or physical and mental distress.

Research shows that patients started on buprenorphine on the spot remain connected with treatment and initially fare far better than those who only get a referral to treatment, which is easy to dismiss. Allowing overdose patients to walk out the door is a missed opportunity. One third of opioid users who overdosed in a year did so again the following year. Half of heroin injectors who survived an overdose will have a fatal overdose at some point. These are scary statistics that further accentuate the need for immediate treatment of overdose victims.

Opportunities to start OUD treatment straightaway really should be endless. Primary care physicians, physician assistants (PAs), and nurse practitioners (NPs) do not need to be addiction experts to offer buprenorphine; they need a short course of training. Professionals throughout the health-care system, however, should have at least a cursory knowledge of OUD as a chronic disorder, understand what evidence-based medical treatments for OUD involve, and be aware of who in the area offers evidence-based treatment.

Addiction treatment centers can also refer stabilized OUD patients to community-based health-care practices. Vermont and Baltimore have successfully implemented this very promising system, sometimes known as hub-and-spoke, and other states have begun to implement it as well. Designed to eliminate wait lists for specialty treatment and reach underserved rural communities, hub-and-spoke systems set up regional outpatient treatment centers (hubs) throughout the state or the city. Staffed by board-certified addiction specialists, hubs are responsible for evaluating patients for OUD and other psychiatric disorders and stabilizing them with medication. Once patients are stabilized, the hub refers them to a spoke, a family doctor in the patient's community who can provide buprenorphine or naltrexone. If patients become unstable, the doctor (spoke) refers them back to the hub. Spokes can consult with hubs and receive ongoing education, which contributes to their proficiency in treating the OUD population.

Training for Medical Providers

Doctors who want to treat OUD patients with buprenorphine need to take an eight-hour course, which can be completed in a one-day training session online or live, or by doing four hours online followed by four hours of live training. PAs and NPs require twenty-four hours of training. Once the session is completed, the provider submits an application and usually receives approval to treat within one to two months. During the first year, providers can prescribe buprenorphine to no more than thirty patients at any time. After one year, the provider can apply to increase the limit of patients to one hundred. After yet another year, physicians who are addiction specialists can apply to have the patient limit increased to 275. To prescribe naltrexone, no training is required. Most providers, however, feel more comfortable after having at least some training and support.

Several high-quality programs, such as Providers' Clinical Support System, offer free training and one-on-one mentoring for medical providers who plan to treat OUD. Medical professionals learn how to evaluate and diagnose OUD, counsel patients about treatment options, initiate treatment, and medically manage those patients. A few online communities for medical providers share information and support colleagues who are new to this area of medical practice. Initial education and support are enough for doctors to become proficient and confident enough to take on more patients.

Steps Leading up to Treatment

Regardless of the setting, treatment usually begins with the patient answering some screening questions. A more detailed assessment and diagnosis based on the American Psychiatric Association's *Diagnostic and Statistical Manual of Mental Disorders (DSM-5)* criteria can come next. Everyone should undergo a brief medical screen to assess any medical or psychiatric concerns. If OUD exists, the provider should offer the patient one of the three medications approved by the FDA for use in treating OUD.

Screening: Screening individuals for opioid and other substance use disorders can take place in a doctor's office, the emergency room, school, prison, or a social services setting. Routine screening can pinpoint individuals who have experienced problems because of substance use (such as a DUI) or already developed a substance use disorder. Professionals have access to several useful screening questionnaires that patients can complete in a matter of minutes. A frequently used questionnaire is the Drug Abuse Screening Tool (DAST-10), which asks ten simple yes/no questions, such as "Are you always able to stop using drugs when you want to?" Answers are more likely to be accurate if the screener ensures confidentiality.

Brief intervention: When screening reveals problems related to substance use, the screener has an opportunity to discuss those problems openly with the patient. This intervention is part of the SBIRT approach described in chapter 3. The session can be brief, lasting as little as five to ten minutes. The focus is on educating patients about the risks of substance use, without judgment or confrontation, and allowing patients to tell their part of the story and to disagree. With patients who are at risk, the screener ends the meeting with positive feedback and appeals to patients' values (for instance, wanting to be fit or respected by their children) with a suggestion to consider drinking or using less, preferably with a specific goal (for example, no more than four drinks per night, two nights per week, for a man). The patient can then schedule a follow-up appointment to review those goals in three or four weeks.

If the patient has a significant problem related to drug use, perhaps a substance use disorder, the screener immediately refers the patient for further evaluation and treatment with a medical provider. Not all patients are motivated, so the screener can use techniques proven to increase follow-through with the referral: make the phone call with the patient and set up the appointment at that moment; make frequent follow-up phone calls until the first meeting with a new provider takes place; and involve a significant other, friend, or a patient navigator who can accompany the patient to the evaluation. If trained to provide a more detailed addiction evaluation, the provider can offer treatment on the spot.

Evaluation: An evaluation involves testing for opioids and any other substances in the body and asking about symptoms of opioid withdrawal to confirm physical dependence. Equally important are the patient's medical and psychological health, motivation to begin treatment, and goals (what does the patient want?). Finally, the provider takes this time to establish a therapeutic relationship with the patient based on trust and respect.

Medical and/or psychiatric evaluation: Acute medical problems, such as confusion, unresponsiveness, fever, or seizures, as well as serious psychiatric conditions, such as psychosis or suicidality, should be addressed before a person begins treatment. Other mental health issues can be addressed at the same time as addiction is treated, preferably in a setting that treats coexisting disorders. (See pages 116–124 for more about treating co-occurring disorders.)

Diagnosis: Diagnosis always comes before prescribing medication, although in urgent cases, a full, Rolls-Royce assessment can come after treatment is started. Professionals rely on the *DSM-5* for a list of OUD symptoms, which include cravings to use drugs, failure to stop or reduce drug use, spending a lot of time using and obtaining large amounts of drugs, continuing use despite problems with health or responsibilities, and finally, the presence of drug tolerance or withdrawal symptoms (see a list of diagnostic standards on page 60). The patient can have mild, moderate, or severe OUD depending on how many criteria they meet.

Education: Patients have a right to be fully educated about treatment options. Providers should explain the three main medications used to treat OUD and cover requirements to start treatment; advantages and limitations of each option; side effects and other risks, including overdose and dropout issues; and duration of treatment for each medication. Providers should also explain the different treatment settings: inpatient units, residential programs, outpatient specialized programs, and treatment at a community health clinic with a primary care doctor. The importance of specialized behavioral approaches, self-help groups, and recovery-oriented activities should be part of the discussion as well. Finally, the patient should thoroughly understand the risks of delaying treatment and the risk of treatment without medication. Providers should inform all patients diagnosed with OUD that they have a chronic disorder that will most likely progress if left untreated and that may result in irreversible complications and even death.

Decision-making: At this point, patients have to make a decision, and they should have all the information needed to evaluate their options and to choose treatment in collaboration with their doctor. Providers need to review access to treatment in the patient's community and cost. Patients should be given time to think over the decision and ask questions. When available and appropriate, the final discussion should involve a family member or a significant other.

Long-Term Treatment: One Size Does Not Fit All

OUD, like many other disorders, is chronic. The word *cure* is never used, because the changes in the brain persist, and relapse is always a possibility. When relapse occurs, the brain pathways involved in maintaining a repetitive opioid use reactivate rapidly. Cravings, tolerance, and physical dependence increase accordingly. The goals of treating OUD are the same as they are for other chronic medical or psychiatric illnesses. Medical professionals work to: (1) reduce the severity of symptoms to nonproblematic levels; (2) improve physical health and psychological well-being; (3) improve functioning and quality of life; and (4) teach patients to monitor their disorder, identify threats to relapse, and become responsible for managing their disorder. *All four goals are achieved much more quickly if medication is begun as soon as possible.*

Not everyone responds the same way to a method of treatment, and anyone charged with determining how a person with OUD should be treated has a responsibility to inform the patient about all the available options—including treatment without medication. Yet this rarely happens. Different treatment centers prefer one form of treatment over another. They create treatment silos. Some, for instance, prefer naltrexone over buprenorphine or methadone over naltrexone. In addition, providers need to expose patients to different aspects of treatment, when needed. Many patients need more than medication.

Evidence-based treatment for OUD involves a combination of several approaches:

- *Medication-assisted treatment (MAT)*—involves the use of medications, usually in combination with an intervention to increase adherence to medications
- *Psychosocial/behavioral approach*—focuses on helping patients develop the skills necessary to cope with cravings and life stressors without drugs
- *Self-help/mutual support groups*—encourages participation in support groups or forming a social network of people supportive of recovery
- *Recovery-oriented activities*—helps patients develop productive and satisfying lives

Once a patient is stabilized, providers can individualize a range of possible treatment goals for each patient. The ultimate goal is to initiate long-term recovery, which the Betty Ford Institute Consensus Panel in 2017 defined as "[a] voluntarily maintained lifestyle characterized by sobriety, personal health, and citizenship."

The New Definition of Sobriety

The traditional definition of sobriety is being free of all mood-altering substances. The opioid epidemic has changed the definition of sobriety. Many addiction professionals now agree that people treated with methadone or buprenorphine (both opioids), as well as naltrexone, are sober, provided they abstain from alcohol and other drugs.

Medication with psychosocial treatment (counseling and behavioral therapy) and mutual support groups is a powerhouse treatment for OUD. The medication can reduce physical discomfort, improve mood, and eliminate cravings for opioids, all of which helps to prevent relapse—the number one life-saving goal for people with OUD. The three FDA-approved medications proven to help treat OUD are methadone, buprenorphine, and naltrexone. Understanding how they work, how they differ, and which is most appropriate for any given individual is important when deciding on a treatment plan. Prescribers, patients, and family members who understand the pharmacology can avoid making some common mistakes.

CHAPTER 5

The Pharmacology of Opioids

Our understanding of how opioid addiction works in the brain began with the search for the Holy Grail of pharmaceuticals: a nonaddictive painkiller stronger than aspirin or Tylenol. In the 1970s, researchers in Scotland first isolated endorphins (meaning "morphine-like"), the body's natural painkillers. Suddenly, we could start exploring how endorphin-like substances produced in the body and those coming from the outside affect brain function to make us feel so good.

Endorphins are the body's natural painkillers and stress reducers. We release endorphins when we exercise (think of the "runner's high") or have sex. Even certain foods trigger a release of endorphins. Like heroin or prescription painkillers, endorphins latch onto a cell's opioid receptors and activate a cascade of chemical events inside the cell. We now know that the body naturally produces a lot of different opioids, beyond endorphins, to regulate various functions. To respond to these natural opioids, the body evolved a large number of different opioid receptor sites spread throughout various organs, primarily the brain and the gut.

Opioid receptor sites are part of the communication network within and between body organs. Most receptor sites are located on nerve cells designed to bind chemicals released into the blood or brain tissue. The entire opioid receptor system plays an important role in regulating the development and functioning of humans and all vertebrate animals; for example, it helps regulate social behavior by decreasing stress and aggression.

One type of opioid receptor is called "mu" (the Greek letter for "*m*"). It was named for morphine, the first substance found to attach to this type of site. Most of the therapeutic effects of the FDA-approved medications (buprenorphine, methadone, and naltrexone) used to treat opioid use disorder (OUD) can link to a mu receptor. While each of the medications has a unique mechanism of action, all of them attach to the same type of opioid receptor sites on the nerve cells. Painkillers and illicit opioids also attach to the mu opioid receptors. For simplicity's sake, I will refer to all such substances, whether therapeutic medication or illicit substances, as "drugs."

What Happens to the Drug in the Body

All opioid drugs have similar effects on the body and brain. There is little difference in how heroin and oxycodone activate opioid receptors, for instance. However, there are differences between the drugs that make some of them addictive, others excellent as medication, and still others that can be both, depending on how they are used. Four important characteristics of drugs help determine whether they are harmful or helpful for someone addicted to opioids:

- How quickly the drug enters your brain
- How long the medication stays active in your body
- How strongly the drug binds (attaches) to the receptor
- How much the medication activates the receptor

How quickly the drug enters your brain

When you take a drug, your blood absorbs and then distributes it to your brain and other organs. The drug then finds its way to your nerve cells and receptors within the organs. How much effect it has depends in part on how fast the drug enters your brain—the organ responsible for producing the high. The more receptors the drug attaches to at once, the stronger the effect. For example, injecting heroin into a vein floods your brain in less than a minute, creating a powerful euphoric effect. The same happens if you inhale a drug deep into your lungs (which happens with smoking), as it mixes directly with blood vessels in the lungs. It takes a bit longer for the drug to reach the brain if you inject it under your skin (skin popping) or into the muscle, but the high still comes on in a matter of a few minutes. Drugs taken nasally (snorted or sniffed) enter your blood through an area of your nose heavily populated with blood vessels, which carry the drug directly to your brain, though some of the drug gets swallowed. It takes a few minutes, but delivery is still fast. When you swallow a pill, it first moves through your esophagus and stomach to the intestines, where it is absorbed into your blood system. The blood flows directly to your liver, where some of the drug is inactivated (metabolized), but some will still manage to reach your brain. Drugs taken orally may take one or more hours to have an effect, and the impact is not usually as strong as with the other routes.

How long the medication stays active in your body

Once the drug is distributed throughout your body, however it entered initially, it goes with the blood to your liver, where it gradually becomes inactivated and later eliminated from your body in urine or feces. Some drugs are inactivated and eliminated very quickly, in a matter of hours, but some linger and remain active for several days. For example, naloxone, a medicine used to reverse opioid overdose, works for only thirty minutes and is eliminated in one to two hours, whereas buprenorphine works for six to twenty-four hours. Some of buprenorphine's effects last longer than others; for example, it blocks withdrawal symptoms for a protracted period but does not work as long to reduce pain. Buprenorphine may take three to four days before it leaves your body—and even longer if it is taken over an extended period of time. The longer a drug remains in your system, the more likely it is to find its way to the receptor and the more stubbornly it will cling to it.

How strongly the drug binds (attaches) to the receptor

A drug can attach to a receptor with a low, medium, or strong bind. The stronger the bind, or the more "sticky" the drug is, the more difficult it is for another substance to "push it off" the receptor. The stronger the bond, the more dominant the effect of the drug when other drugs are also present. If more than one opioid drug is present, they "compete" for the receptor site. Drugs that have quantity *and* a stronger bind in their favor dominate.

How much the medication activates the receptor

Drugs are classified depending on the type of effect they produce at the receptor site. Once attached to the receptor, the drug can activate it a little, a lot, or not at all. Those that activate the receptor are known as agonists and those that do not are known as antagonists.

Full agonists attach to a receptor and activate it to the fullest extent possible. The more drug molecules present in your brain, the greater the effect. Think of full agonists as a gas pedal on a car: The more the gas pedal is pressed, the faster the car goes. Morphine, heroin, fentanyl, oxycodone, and methadone are full agonists.

Partial agonists attach to the receptor but have only about 50 percent of the effect of a full agonist. Partial agonists have a ceiling effect; that is, once that partial effect is reached, introducing more drug molecules has no effect. Partial agonists are like a car built with a limit on the acceleration: Initially, the more the gas pedal is pressed, the faster the car goes, but once it reaches a certain speed, it cannot go any faster, even if the gas pedal is pressed more. Buprenorphine is a partial agonist. Its ceiling effect is important for safety. Unlike full agonists, buprenorphine is unable to completely shut down the breathing center in your brain, which is what happens during an opioid overdose, even if the medication activates all receptors. Overdose can occur in children, however, or if the drug is combined with high doses of another sedative medication, such as alprazolam (Xanax).

Antagonists attach to the receptor but produce no activation, regardless of the amount of drug present. It is like a car with a disconnected fuel line: No matter how much the gas pedal is pressed, it has no effect on the car's speed. The medications naloxone and naltrexone are opioid antagonists.

How Medication Interacts with Heroin or Painkillers

Heroin, prescription painkillers, methadone, buprenorphine, and naltrexone will compete for opioid receptors. The "winner," or whichever drug is the pushiest, dominates. Understanding this phenomenon is important before we consider how each individual treatment is best prescribed. Most people who start treatment often have more than one of these substances in their body, and some of those individuals will use while on medication. Explaining what happens when these drugs interact can eliminate unpleasant surprises and improve the treatment experience. Here are the most common scenarios (note that heroin and painkillers have an almost equal effect on receptor sites):

Methadone and heroin/painkillers have about the same level of receptor activation, but methadone has a stronger bind with the receptor than heroin. If both are present, methadone will force heroin out of a receptor, yet there is little to no change in how you feel. You will feel "normal" provided the concentration of methadone remains stable compared to the usual heroin intake. If you use heroin while you are being treated with methadone, the heroin will struggle to dislodge the methadone, in addition to the high tolerance, so the effects of the heroin will be partially blocked. High doses of heroin, however, can overpower methadone.

Buprenorphine and heroin/painkillers both activate receptors, but buprenorphine is a partial agonist. It will produce half of the effect that heroin can produce. Buprenorphine, however, has a stronger receptor binding that heroin or methadone. Therefore, if you have a lot of heroin in your system, fully activating many receptors, bringing buprenorphine on board will push the heroin off the receptors and abruptly decrease the activation of the receptors by half. Within a matter of minutes, you will feel different—the heroin-produced euphoria will disappear, and you will go into withdrawal. The fact that buprenorphine can push heroin off receptors while decreasing receptor activation might be why we hear reports of heroin overdoses that were reversed with buprenorphine, though use of buprenorphine for this purpose has not been studied.

If you are using heroin (or being treated with methadone) and you do not take the next dose at the usual time, the heroin comes off the receptors and is gradually eliminated from your body. This will trigger opioid withdrawal, which increases in severity as more receptors become vacant. If buprenorphine is then added, it attaches to and starts activating the receptors, which helps eliminate withdrawal. The "partial effect" of buprenorphine is sufficient to fully eliminate withdrawal, but the medication will not produce euphoria (full receptor activation is needed for the latter). This period of mild withdrawal is necessary if you are a heroin user taking your first dose of buprenorphine or if you transition from treatment with methadone onto treatment with buprenorphine.

Once you take buprenorphine every day as a medicine, it "sticks" to the receptors quite hard, and an "average" dose of heroin has difficulty getting onto the receptors. Buprenorphine will block a lot of heroin's effects. Because it "sticks" hard, it is a better blocker of heroin than methadone is.

Naltrexone and heroin/painkillers have the opposite effect on opioid receptors. Heroin fully activates them and naltrexone stimulates no activity. Naltrexone "blocks" the receptor. Because naltrexone binds to the receptor quite strongly, it averts other drugs (heroin, painkillers, methadone, buprenorphine) from getting on and activating receptors. If you have a lot of heroin, methadone, or buprenorphine in your system, are physically dependent on it, and then take naltrexone, the naltrexone shoves the agonists off the receptors and suddenly the whole opioid system goes from full speed to an abrupt stop: Your body goes into sudden and severe "precipitated" withdrawal as soon as naltrexone reaches enough of the opioid receptors in your brain (in one to two hours). This severe withdrawal can last many hours. And naltrexone can precipitate withdrawal even several days after you take the last dose of an opioid agonist.

Precipitated withdrawal, which is for many people unbearable, can also be dangerous because it can produce excessive fluid in your lungs or seizures. To avoid precipitated withdrawal, you must go through a detoxification, or a "washout" period, before safely starting treatment with naltrexone. The washout period can be shortened by starting naltrexone with very small doses (but such small doses are not yet commercially available). These cautions aside, taken regularly, naltrexone capably blocks most opioid receptors. Heroin, but also methadone and buprenorphine, if taken in usual doses, will not produce any effects in a person treated with naltrexone.

Naloxone and heroin/painkillers interact the same way naltrexone and heroin do, except your body rapidly neutralizes naloxone. Naloxone is therefore a good choice for reversing opioid overdose. Naloxone hustles to reach the receptors and at once jolts excessive amounts of heroin off the receptors to quickly restore respiration in the event of an overdose. The effects of naloxone, however, disappear in a half hour, whereas those of heroin persist for many hours. Unless naloxone is given repeatedly, you will overdose again from the opioids still in your body. If the dose of naloxone is too high, your body will become alert and then go into a precipitated withdrawal. Therefore, naloxone should be given in small, repeated doses and closely monitored. For that reason, anyone who administers naloxone outside of a medical setting needs to call 911 and arrange for transport to a hospital.

The "blocking" effect of naltrexone, methadone, and buprenorphine is relative, not absolute. A high enough dose of heroin or fentanyl can overpower the "blockade" and result in an overdose. This is rare but possible if you are on medication and you try to take a large enough dose of heroin to "override" the medication blockade. Overdoses usually occur if you decide to stop taking medication and resume heroin or fentanyl use.

Buprenorphine versus buprenorphine with naloxone: Buprenorphine is a partial agonist, whereas naloxone is a short-acting antagonist. Most of the products containing buprenorphine also include naloxone (these are known as "buprenorphine combination products"; e.g., Suboxone and Zubsolv). The main reason for adding naloxone is to reduce the abuse potential of buprenorphine in case it is injected. When taken together sublingually (i.e., beneath the tongue, which is how it is prescribed), most of the naloxone is rapidly inactivated while the buprenorphine is absorbed and remains active. When buprenorphine and naloxone are taken together by injection or by snorting, the naloxone remains active and blocks some of the effect of the buprenorphine. When buprenorphine, with or without naloxone, is injected or snorted by a daily user of heroin or painkillers, it will precipitate withdrawal because it pushes the heroin off the receptors and brings down the activation of the receptor from 100 to 50 percent; however, if injected by a person who is taking only buprenorphine, it will not precipitate withdrawal but produce euphoria (it will not change the level of the receptor activation, which stays at 50 percent). The addition of naloxone in buprenorphine products reduces the euphoric effects and abuse potential of buprenorphine, but does not eliminate them.

Using Medications in Treatment

Methadone has been used clinically since the 1960s. It was the first medication approved to treat OUD. It is a full mu opioid receptor agonist with a medium receptor-binding strength with properties that make it a good medication choice. Methadone is available as a solution, usually dispensed in opioid treatment programs, or as a tablet, which is used for the treatment of pain. Methadone is taken by mouth, and its effects come on very gradually and persist for a long time, usually for twenty-four hours, just in time for your next daily dose. With a proper dosing of methadone, there is little variation in the stimulation of opioid receptors. You do not experience drug intoxication (seen when blood level of the drug is rising rapidly) or withdrawal (seen when blood level of the drug is decreasing). The consistent activation of the opioid system prevents the development of opioid withdrawal if you are reducing or stopping heroin. This helps you further reduce your heroin use and stop it completely without risking the distress of opioid withdrawal.

Methadone's consistent, medium-level stimulation of the opioid system prevents ups and downs of receptor activation. Therefore, properly administered methadone stabilizes the functioning of the opioid system, and with that it decreases pathological brain responses to drug cues and stress. This effect contributes to the reduction or total elimination of craving for heroin, which helps put an end to heroin consumption. Stabilization of the opioid system also appears to have added benefits. Mood is more constant and anxiety and depression reduced, all of which further helps improve well-being.

Constant stimulation of opioid receptors with sufficient doses of methadone also induces a high level of tolerance, which is a protective measure against strong receptor activation. Tolerance decreases the sensitivity of your brain to opioids, similar to turning down the gain on a microphone. Because people being treated with methadone have a high level of opioid tolerance, those who continue to have urges and use heroin experience very little euphoria. Methadone can "block" the effects of heroin by maintaining high tolerance and directly competing for receptor sites with heroin. As a result, most individuals do not experience an increase in craving and do not escalate heroin use, and many eventually stop using altogether.

Heroin-Assisted Treatment

An emerging treatment for longtime, severe OUD is heroin-assisted treatment (HAT). Developed and first used in Switzerland, HAT follows in the same vein as the narcotic clinics that existed at the beginning of the twentieth century. Heroin users receive controlled doses of pharmacological heroin—heroin produced in a laboratory rather than bought off the street—in a monitored setting. HAT is now used in several European countries as well as in Canada, primarily for heroin users who did not do well in methadone programs. The results are promising: improved health, stabilized dosages, significantly reduced illicit drug use, and a major reduction in criminal activity.

Buprenorphine has been in use as a pain medicine since the early 1980s, and in 2002 the FDA approved its use in the treatment of opioid dependence. Buprenorphine is a partial agonist of the mu opioid receptors with a medium-high receptor binding strength. It also attaches to other opioid receptor sites, which may explain its ability to enhance mood and diminish craving. Because buprenorphine acts as an agonist, it shares many of the same beneficial effects of methadone.

Buprenorphine is generally not taken by mouth because if swallowed, close to 90 percent becomes inactivated in your liver before it has a chance to reach your brain. Sublingual buprenorphine preparations are designed to be absorbed by your body directly through the lining of your mouth (mucosa). You place the tablet or the film under your tongue or against the inside of your cheek and leave it there until it completely dissolves, without swallowing if possible. With sublingual preparations, approximately 30 to 40 percent of the medication is absorbed, though this percentage varies from person to person. The effects of buprenorphine last for one to two days. With higher doses (32 mg or greater), there is enough active medication to produce an effect for two to three days, so it can be given every other day. Lower doses (less than 2 mg) wear off fast and may need to be taken twice per day to prevent withdrawal symptoms.

Buprenorphine is also available as an injection or as an implant. In both cases, a large amount of the medicine is placed under your skin, and your body slowly absorbs close to 100 percent of it. Therefore, you can receive a buprenorphine injection up to once per month, and a buprenorphine implant lasts up to six months. Buprenorphine is also available as a low-dose skin patch for pain, but this form is not approved to treat OUD.

When taken as prescribed and in appropriate doses, buprenorphine continually activates the opioid system without producing euphoria or withdrawal. This effect is similar to what we see with methadone. However, because buprenorphine produces less receptor activation than methadone, the effects are even less perceptible than with methadone. Most people do not feel much different after they take their dose, or even if they delay taking their dose.

Similarly to methadone, the constant activation of opioid receptors prevents opioid withdrawal after heroin is stopped and stabilizes the functioning of the opioid system. This reduces opioid craving. Individuals treated with buprenorphine also report improved mood and sleep and feeling "clear-headed." Elimination of withdrawal and craving, along with improved mood, is enough to lead many people to stop using heroin or painkillers. Buprenorphine forms a strong bind with the opioid receptors. It effectively blocks heroin, which prevents escalation of use in those who continue to crave and use heroin while taking their daily dose of buprenorphine.

Naltrexone has been used in treatment of OUD since the early 1970s, first as a daily tablet. In 2010, the FDA approved a monthly injection for treatment of OUD. Naltrexone is an antagonist of the mu opioid receptors with a high receptor-binding strength. People can swallow naltrexone tablets to absorb approximately 25 percent of the medication. A standard 50 mg dose remains active, blocking opioid receptors for up to two days. Because of the long-lasting effect, naltrexone can be given in a higher dose (100–150 mg) every two or three days. A slow-release injection, which has enough medication (380 mg) to last up to four weeks, ensures that close to 100 percent of it is absorbed. Naltrexone is also available as an implant, surgically placed under the skin, with effects lasting up to six months. This preparation is approved in Russia but not in the United States, as there is very limited research on its safety and the duration of its effects.

It is important to note that naltrexone can only be started in individuals who have completed opioid withdrawal and remained abstinent from opioids for at least several days. If given too soon after the last opioid dose, the medication may precipitate withdrawal. Once naltrexone is started, however, it can be continued without concern about withdrawal. Even if the person occasionally uses heroin (to no effect), it is unlikely that physical dependence will be reestablished if naltrexone is continued at therapeutic doses, and additional naltrexone will not produce withdrawal.

Naltrexone stabilizes the opioid receptor system by "turning it down." The continued blockade of opioid receptors eliminates the possibility of opioid euphoria and withdrawal. Craving for opioids is reduced or eliminated and mood improved in many people treated with naltrexone. All these positive effects of naltrexone encourage abstinence. Additionally, naltrexone acts as a well-buttressed wall against all opioids, because it forms a strong bind with opioid receptors. Therefore, people who continue to have urges and use heroin do not experience any effects and usually do not escalate their use. Somewhat surprisingly, naltrexone does not seem to shut off opioid receptor sites activated by the body's naturally occurring opioids, such as endorphins. Most of the known functions supported by natural opioids seem to be unaffected by the presence of naltrexone, most likely because there are many different types of opioid receptors and the opioid system adapts well to change.

Medication Treatment Outcomes

Methadone is used worldwide and included on the World Health Organization's (WHO) Model List of Essential Medicines, a compilation of medications that are effective, safe, affordable, and recommended for use in health-care systems globally. Methadone is one of the most studied medications in the whole of medicine, and most studies show that methadone is superior when compared to treatment without any medication. People treated with methadone experience marked reductions of heroin and other drug use and stay in treatment longer; as a result, they live longer and have fewer medical problems when compared to those with OUD who are not treated with methadone. Moreover, some studies show reduction in injections and other drug-related HIV risk behavior, lower rates of crime, and improved social and work functioning among individuals treated with methadone.

Methadone is the most effective of all treatment approaches, reducing overdoses by at least half. Under optimal conditions, 75 percent of those who start methadone remain in treatment for at least six months, and most experience significant benefits from treatment. The longer they stay in treatment, the more benefits they experience. The average dose of methadone should be in the range of 60 to 120 mg/day, and higher doses are more effective than lower doses.

Buprenorphine is also used in many countries around the world and has been added, alongside methadone, to the WHO Model List of Essential Medicines. The safety and effectiveness of buprenorphine has been studied extensively, although less than methadone. Most studies show benefits similar to methadone, primarily reduction of illicit opioid use and longer stays in treatment. Buprenorphine may also help reduce the use of other drugs.

On average, 50 percent of people on buprenorphine remain in treatment for at least six months and continue to experience treatment benefits. As with methadone, the benefits of buprenorphine continue as long as the person is maintained on the medication. The usual dose of buprenorphine used for maintenance is 8 to 24 mg/day, and similarly to methadone, higher doses of buprenorphine are more effective than lower doses. Because buprenorphine is a partial agonist, it is thought that doses higher than 32 mg a day do not offer any additional benefits. The most common reason the medication is not effective is that the individual being treated is not fully adherent to the prescribed dosage.

When compared to methadone, those treated with buprenorphine have less reduction in opioid use and lower participation in treatment. Methadone is likely more effective because it produces stronger opioid effects, which may be necessary for some people to fully benefit from treatment. On the other hand, buprenorphine is a safer medication, with less risk of side effects and adverse effects, including a lower risk of death from overdose.

Naltrexone in tablet form was at at first found mostly effective in a small group of people who would have significant external negative consequences if they did not continue with medications, such as physicians who could lose their licenses to practice or parolees who would be returned to prison if they relapsed. Most of those who received the tablets did not like taking naltrexone because they had to suffer through withdrawal first and did not feel well for several weeks; in consequence, most stopped taking it as soon as they had a chance. The introduction of long-acting, extended-release (XR-) naltrexone in 2010 has increased naltrexone's popularity and reduced early treatment dropout rates. Receiving an injection with enough naltrexone to last a month helps people to continue benefiting from the medication when they do not feel well: After the first few weeks, most feel much better and are willing to take additional doses of naltrexone. Treatment with naltrexone injections doubles the rate of individuals remaining abstinent and in treatment at six months as compared to treatment with daily naltrexone tablets. The naltrexone implant, when it becomes available in the United States, may even further reduce treatment dropout.

When started after detoxification, XR-naltrexone helps people remain abstinent and stay in treatment as compared to treatment without naltrexone. Up to 50 percent of those treated with XR-naltrexone injections remain in treatment and free of relapse at six months. However, it is more difficult to start treatment with XR-naltrexone than it is to start treatment with buprenorphine: About 30 to 40 percent of individuals who are actively using opioids cannot start XR-naltrexone, as compared to 5 percent who cannot start buprenorphine. But among those who receive the first dose, rates of success are comparable to those treated with buprenorphine. As with buprenorphine and methadone, stopping treatment early—for example, after only six months—leaves many people at risk of relapse.

Limitations of Treatment with Medications

The potential of the medications used to treat OUD goes well beyond current outcomes. Methadone, buprenorphine, and naltrexone are limited by some very preventable or changeable circumstances: (1) Much of the public does not know enough about these medications and the need for chronic treatment. (2) Prescribers tend to dose too low or fail to adequately address co-occurring psychiatric disorders. (3) Recipients are misled by providers, family members, or their own thinking to prematurely discontinue medication, or they use other drugs in addition to their prescribed treatment. Other limitations, specific to each drug, are harder to overcome:

Methadone and buprenorphine

Methadone and buprenorphine are controlled substances. Multiple government agencies oversee the distribution of methadone. The highly restricted drug is only available in specialized treatment centers, now called opioid treatment programs, or OTPs (formerly referred to as methadone maintenance programs). Methadone treatment is highly structured, and the prescribing physician has little flexibility. The FDA also regulates treatment with buprenorphine, but physicians have much more flexibility in terms of dosage, number of doses given, and frequency of monitoring.

Methadone is a potent opioid agonist and, if used inappropriately, can produce sedation or even overdose and death, which is one of the reasons treatment with methadone needs to be closely monitored. This risk is the greatest during treatment initiation and after treatment termination or dropout. Buprenorphine is much safer. The risk of excessive sedation or overdose is very low.

People can misuse either medication to achieve euphoria. The most common method is to inject the substance into a vein. To reduce this risk, methadone is given under observation, and take-home doses are given as a large-volume flavored solution, which stops most recipients from injecting it but not from doubling up or giving it to someone else. Buprenorphine is usually combined with naloxone, which reduces the risk of abuse, although it does not eliminate it (see page 93).

As with any controlled substance, diversion of methadone and buprenorphine is an issue. Both medicines can be illegally rerouted to people who do not have a prescription. Most often, diverted medication is used "therapeutically" by others who take it to decrease withdrawal, craving, and opioid use. But there is nothing to stop people for whom they are prescribed from selling these medications on the black market and snatching the profits to buy heroin or other drugs, which clearly undermines the benefits of medication treatment.

Diversion-Reduction Plan

Providers can institute diversion-reduction plans as an essential part of treatment with buprenorphine. Diversion-reduction plans include:

- Frequent urine tests to confirm that buprenorphine is taken as prescribed
- A pill count at each visit to make sure the right amount of the medication is left over
- Random callbacks to the office between scheduled visits for additional urine tests and pill counts
- A limited supply of medication (for example, someone treated with a high dosage may receive a weekly rather than monthly supply at a time)
- Supervised administration of medication either in the clinic or at home with a significant other

The pervasive stigma associated with such medications as methadone or buprenorphine makes it difficult for people to enter, accept, and remain in treatment over the long term. Young individuals in particular find it burdensome to think of themselves as needing long-term treatment. Finally, integrating methadone or buprenorphine with mainstream recovery-oriented self-help support groups such as Narcotics Anonymous is challenging, as many members of these groups view medication as the antithesis of recovery.

Naltrexone

Availability of naltrexone is more limited than buprenorphine due to its novelty. Individuals who are actively using opioids and want to start naltrexone need to be admitted to a program or work with a provider who can manage the detoxification and induction. The best venue is an inpatient unit, where the person can undergo a medically supervised withdrawal and is not able to act on cravings to use. But many inpatient programs do not yet offer naltrexone following detoxification.

Naltrexone is a potent opioid blocker, and those maintained on naltrexone are not able to benefit from standard opioid-based treatment for pain. Other strategies can be used under the supervision of a pain specialist, but the idea of not being able to relieve pain with opioids is frightening for many for whom pain is a consideration.

Diverting naltrexone pills is a nonissue because naltrexone is not a controlled substance and has no "street" value. People can only receive a naltrexone injection in the doctor's office, so adherence is 100 percent guaranteed provided they come to their appointment on time.

Medication-Assisted Treatment: Using Medications in Combination with Psychosocial Treatments

For the best outcomes, we need to monitor and support those in recovery from opioid addiction over the long term. The best way to achieve this is to combine medication with psychosocial interventions designed to work in tune with the medication. This combination approach improves outcomes in a way not possible when these treatments are given in isolation. With OUD the scales are tipped somewhat: The effect of medication alone is much stronger than the effect of psychosocial treatment alone.

Regardless, writing a prescription without asking how the patient is using the medication and without troubleshooting problems related to the use of the medication is often ineffective and substandard. Physicians are used to the *medical management model* used in treatment of other chronic disorders. This approach involves periodic face-to-face visits when a prescription needs to be renewed. The provider reevaluates the patient's physical and psychological functioning, medication adherence, and the medication's beneficial effects and side effects. Medical management is often not considered a psychosocial approach because it is done by a medical provider, though it certainly has elements of such. The medical management model can be very effective when used to deliver treatment with buprenorphine or XR-naltrexone, even without additional psychosocial or behavioral interventions.

Psychosocial treatments and behavioral treatments are interventions that use psychological rather than biological means. The terms are often used interchangeably, though *behavioral interventions* aim to change patients' behavior, whereas the more general *psychosocial interventions* aim to produce a change in people's symptoms, functioning, and well-being. For example, behavioral interventions may include setting up positive or negative consequences for a specific behavior, whereas a psychosocial intervention may include identifying triggers that increase drug craving. The overall purpose of these interventions is to improve quality of life so that individuals are more likely to follow their treatment plans and stay off drugs that could derail their success. Psychosocial treatments include education about their disorder; evidence-based psychotherapy; and case management, which is a service that helps people solve problems that prevent them from meeting their social and health needs.

CHAPTER 6

Starting a Patient on Medication

Treatment with medications should be offered to all people with opioid use disorder (OUD), whether the disorder is mild, moderate, or severe; current, or in a partial or full remission. This includes those who are actively using opioids at the time of the evaluation; those who have never developed a daily routine of opioid use but suffer from adverse consequences of occasional use; those who recently stopped daily use of opioids and are not physically dependent at the time of evaluation; and those who have remained abstinent for some time but may have a recurrence of cravings or simply undergo additional stress or problems in their lives.

OUD is a chronic disorder, and once it develops it remains present whether the patient is using or not. Use is just one of the disorder's many hallmarks. People who have recently become abstinent after undergoing full opioid withdrawal (detoxification) or who are not taking any opioids (heroin, fentanyl, painkillers, methadone, buprenorphine) and do not have any signs of opioid withdrawal are not physically dependent. However, all of them still have a disorder that requires treatment. The first decision health-care professionals must make about the choice of medication depends on whether a person with OUD is physically dependent at the beginning of treatment.

Patients Who Are Not Physically Dependent

Patients with OUD who are not physically dependent include those who have recently become abstinent on their own at home and those just leaving a controlled environment, such as a residential program or jail. These people have a high risk of relapse and overdose if they remain untreated. Patients who are not physically dependent at the time of evaluation have the option of initiating treatment with naltrexone as a relapse prevention strategy or treatment with buprenorphine (see table, p. 110). Patients may choose between naltrexone tablets or a monthly naltrexone injection.

Patients can take naltrexone tablets on their own or with the supervision of a significant other. Some patients can even take a naltrexone tablet as needed—for example, when anticipating increased stress or risk of cravings to use, such as before weekends or an event where drugs and drug-using friends might be present. Patients may also take naltrexone when they begin experiencing craving. The option to take naltrexone tablets as needed leaves a lot of flexibility, which is attractive to some people, especially those who have a history of remaining abstinent for long periods of time. However, patients who become ambivalent about abstinence can easily stop taking tablets and relapse, so this is not an option for those who are just beginning treatment. Patients who are abstinent may benefit greatly from ongoing contact with a therapist, either individually or in a group setting, to take advantage of monitoring and develop skills to minimize the risk of relapse.

An even more effective relapse prevention strategy is for patients to receive ongoing injections of long-acting naltrexone. Many patients have a hard time predicting when they may have urges to use or forgo taking medication once the urges set in. Physicians should offer those who are leaving controlled settings and returning to high-risk environments the naltrexone injection. Tablets are unlikely to adequately protect patients at high risk of medication nonadherence.

An alternative for patients at high risk of relapse is treatment with buprenorphine, given daily as a maintenance strategy, which can be very effective in reducing cravings. However, these patients need to understand that once they begin daily use of buprenorphine, they will be physically dependent on opioids, which in itself is not a major issue as long as they continue taking the medication as prescribed. Some patients and their families may feel uneasy about being physically dependent on the medication and risking withdrawal. Yet many medications used on a chronic basis produce physical adaptations and symptoms of withdrawal if abruptly stopped, including medications used to treat depression, high blood pressure, and seizures. The fact that medication may produce withdrawal symptoms if abruptly stopped should not by itself be a reason for not starting treatment with medications, especially if the consequences of an untreated disorder can be severe.

Methadone is not usually offered to patients who are able to remain abstinent on their own. Most programs require the presence of a current and active OUD, confirmed with a positive urine test.

Patients Who Are Physically Dependent

Patients who are using opioids daily at the time of the evaluation can start with methadone, buprenorphine, or naltrexone. Those choosing treatment with naltrexone will require detoxification and a period of abstinence before naltrexone can be started; these preliminaries are not necessary if the patient chooses treatment with buprenorphine or methadone. Once the choice is made, the first phase of treatment involves stabilization on the medication, which can take approximately one to two months. During that initial treatment phase, the physician will closely monitor the patient to determine how effective the medication is and whether it is safe and well tolerated. If the patient reports a decrease in craving, no withdrawal symptoms, no opioid use, and no side effects, this is considered a good response. Treatment then enters the maintenance phase, where monitoring is less frequent.

In cases where the patient has some benefits from treatment but continues to struggle, the provider may increase the dose of the medication, offer a different form of the medication, or recommend adding intensive behavioral treatment. If the patient is not able to stabilize within the first few months or has side effects that are difficult to manage, the physician may recommend another medication, either from the same or a different class. For example, patients who start buprenorphine but miss many doses and struggle with frequent cravings and illicit opioid use can try the injection form of buprenorphine, methadone, or detoxification followed by treatment with XR-naltrexone. If treated successfully with methadone, they may transition back to buprenorphine after a period of stability if that is their preference. Likewise, those who respond well to buprenorphine but do not wish to take daily doses may elect a six-month buprenorphine implant. If they want to be off opioid-based medication, they may transition onto XR-naltrexone.

Regardless of the path a patient takes, treatment with medications works best as a maintenance intervention, without a predefined length of treatment. There is no scientific evidence showing benefits to limiting the time someone takes these medications.

Paths to Getting Off Opioids

- Enroll in a methadone program, continue with methadone maintenance
- Enroll in a methadone program, transition onto buprenorphine maintenance
- Initiate buprenorphine, continue with buprenorphine maintenance
- Initiate buprenorphine, go through opioid withdrawal, initiate XR-naltrexone, continue with XR-naltrexone for relapse prevention
- Undergo opioid withdrawal (detoxification) and initiate XR-naltrexone, continue with XR-naltrexone for relapse prevention

Agonist- Versus Antagonist-Based Treatment

One of the most important treatment decisions is choosing between the two main strategies: treatment with an agonist (methadone or buprenorphine) or treatment with an antagonist (naltrexone). The two approaches are very distinct, with different mechanisms of action and different treatment initiation procedures. Neither approach guarantees complete symptom remission, nor is one approach clearly superior. It is difficult to argue that there is one best choice for all patients.

Methadone is considered the gold standard of OUD treatment. While it should be offered and available to all patients, it is not. Many people live too far from opioid treatment programs (OTPs) or can't accept or manage meeting the strict requirements of daily clinic visits in the first months of treatment. Another roadblock is that physicians can only prescribe methadone for OUD if they practice in a registered OTP: Other physicians can prescribe methadone tablets for the treatment of pain but cannot legally prescribe them for OUD. What is clear, however, is that when the choice is individualized—based on a mix of patient preference and the medical provider's recommendation—methadone offers the best chance at the best possible outcome.

Naltrexone may be more appealing to patients uninterested in treatment with opioid agonists, including those working in professions that restrict the use of certain medications. Airline pilots and physicians in some states can lose their licenses if they test positive for opioids, whether prescription or not. Some courts also prohibit people on parole to be treated with agonists. Patients who are detoxified and abstinent for some time may prefer relapse prevention treatment with naltrexone over treatment with an agonist. Those with a less severe form of the disorder and young adults who are unwilling to commit to long-term agonist maintenance may prefer treatment with naltrexone (although it is not known whether naltrexone is more effective in such patients in the long term). Sporadic opioid users and those who are considered high risk—for example, those with a strong family history of OUD and overdose deaths—may opt to be treated with naltrexone as a strategy to protect them from developing a severe disorder or overdosing. Patients who tried agonists previously but were not successful may choose a trial of naltrexone. Finally, those who were successful in treatment with an agonist but wish to discontinue the medication without risking relapse may consider a transition to naltrexone.

Some patients are better candidates for treatment with agonists. Patients with a history of overdoses following detoxification may be particularly vulnerable and should avoid another detoxification and instead seek agonist maintenance. Those with serious medical or psychiatric problems should avoid detoxification, which is usually a stress on the body, and instead stabilize on the agonist. Sometimes an underlying psychiatric disorder becomes unmasked once opioids are taken away, since opioids are well known to have potent antianxiety, antidepressant, and antipsychotic effects.

Choosing Between Buprenorphine and Methadone

Even though treatment with methadone and buprenorphine is somewhat similar, patients and providers need to consider the differences when deciding which medication to use. The effectiveness of each medication is also related to the venue where it is delivered—an OTP in the case of methadone; office-based treatment in the case of buprenorphine. There is also a third, lesser-known option: buprenorphine delivered in the OTP, which is at first given in a very structured way, similar to methadone. Patients who no longer need that structure can take their supply of buprenorphine at home, usually much sooner than is the case with methadone.

Many people may prefer more flexible treatment, with the option to take medication at home. Some prefer the structure and the social component of an OTP, with access to various resources, support groups, and medical care on-site, among other benefits. Physician and patient should consider factors such as ability to adhere to the rules of office-based treatment and follow safety procedures, for example monitoring the medication supply at home. Patients with medical or psychiatric problems, with

Comparison Between Treatment with Methadone/Buprenorphine and Naltrexone

	Methadone or Buprenorphine	Naltrexone
Before starting treatment	Detoxification is not needed.	Detoxification and a washout period are required.
Delay	Treatment can be started with minimal delay.	Delay of 1 to 2 weeks before starting treatment in active opioid users
Physical dependence	Patients remain physically dependent: need to take medication as prescribed, withdrawal symptoms if a dose is delayed or missed.	After detoxification, patients are no longer physically dependent. No opioid withdrawal if medication dose is missed.
Adherence with the medication	Because patients may experience physical discomfort if the dose is delayed, they are more likely to be adherent with the medication.	There is no discomfort if the dose is delayed, and patients may be more likely to stop medication prematurely. This is a major problem with the naltrexone tablet.
Effect on craving	Decreases craving	Decreases craving
Effect on illicit opioid use	Decreases use	Decreases use
Effect on overdose risk	Patients who are adherent with treatment are protected against overdose Increased risk of overdose after treatment dropout and stopping medication	Patients who are adherent with treatment are protected against overdose Increased risk of overdose after treatment dropout and stopping medication Injection naltrexone offers better overdose protection than the tablet form because of better adherence and longer duration of blockade
Potential for abuse and diversion	Can be abused and diverted	None
Overdose risk	When combined with sedatives	None
Side effects during initiation	Sedation, dizziness	Insomnia, diarrhea, low energy, anxiety
Side effects in maintenance phase	Constipation, excessive sweating, injection site reactions	Headache, depression, injection site reactions
Treatment of pain with opioids	Opioid pain medicines can be used	Usual doses of opioid painkillers are not effective, treatment by a pain specialist is needed
Opposition to treatment	Significant stigma against methadone, limited acceptance of agonists in traditional treatment settings Barriers to availability of agonists in criminal justice system	Less stigma against naltrexone in traditional treatment settings
Availability	Limited availability of methadone Better availability of buprenorphine	Very limited availability of injection naltrexone

severe OUD, and those using other substances benefit more from treatment with methadone. Similarly, patients who need additional resources, such as support with housing and employment, may benefit from methadone as compared with buprenorphine.

Predicting how well a patient will do on any given medication can be difficult. Sometimes it is trial and error. Sometimes, though, it works right out of the box.

Nicole's Miracle

After Nicole learns she is pregnant, she tells her doctor she is doing fifteen to twenty bags of heroin a day, plus a gram of coke. This is enough to kill an average person or two, but it does not hurt Nicole or her baby-to-be because she is tolerant to the effects. Her doctor, either not knowing what to do or not realizing it is illegal, puts her on 120 milligrams of oxycodone a day and tapers her off as the weeks go on. This is hard for Nicole. She is going through a slow withdrawal, which probably also affects the development of the fetus. But Nicole thinks of the prize she'll get when she gets through this. Nicole's family has no idea she relapsed after Jake's funeral and used during the first six months of the pregnancy. Nicole has not told them. At this juncture, keeping secrets seems normal.

Robbie is born a robust eight pounds two ounces but suffers from neonatal abstinence syndrome (NAS). He stays in the hospital for four weeks, slowly being weaned from opioids with small drops of morphine, and Nicole is forced to fess up to her family about her use. Her family is heartbroken, but every one of them pitches in to help. Someone is at the hospital with Robbie at all times. He is cuddled, fed, and loved relentlessly. Babies have a way of bringing out the best in everyone, and Robbie is no exception.

Because Nicole has opioids in her system when Robbie is born, even though they are prescription, child protective services opens up a case. Two weeks later, the hospital sends Nicole to detox from oxycodone, and after two days she is sent home with a buprenorphine taper. She is supposed to take half a strip a day for five days. She asks the hospital to keep her longer. "I'm an addict," she pleads. "I can't taper myself. That's why I'm here." But they tell her she will be fine. She knows before she leaves the hospital that the detox was a waste of time. Thoughts of using overpower her. Having a baby she loves and wants to bring home from the hospital is not enough to stop them.

Nicole finishes her five-day supply of buprenorphine in two days and then contacts her dealer. From the moment she starts using heroin, she wants to stop. Nicole lives alone, and her close-knit family has no idea she has relapsed. Forgetting what day it is, Nicole uses heroin first thing in the morning. A call from her mom reminds her that her hearing with a worker from child services is scheduled to take place in a few hours.

Nicole's worst fear is that child protective services will take Robbie and place him in another family, and so she willingly gives her mother custody. For the first year of his life, Robbie is officially raised by Nicole's mom. Nicole is still using but spends most of her time with Robbie. Everyone in the family does whatever they can to help. It is like living in a commune with a revolving door—someone is always coming or going and ready to chip in.

During a session with her therapist, Nicole learns about XR-naltrexone. The thought of a monthly injection appeals to her. And knowing that she would never have to withdraw from the medication is a huge plus. Nicole's therapist refers her to a physician who arranges for her to spend seven days in detox and then administers the drug.

For the first time in about ten years, Nicole has no thoughts of using. Not one. She jokes that the only time she thinks of it is when she wonders why she never thinks about it.

Myths About the Nature
of OUD Treatment

Although medications are very effective in treating even the most severe opioid addiction, they are underused because of some of the myths:

- Opioid addiction is hard to treat. There are no good treatments.
- To receive good treatment, you need to go to a residential program.
- You only need medications for detox, but not to maintain abstinence.
- If you continue medications for too long, you may become addicted to them and will have a hard time getting off them.
- Buprenorphine and methadone work only as replacement drugs. Because these are opioids, you feel their effects and you are still physically dependent on them, which means that you are only trading one addiction for another.
- Buprenorphine and methadone are more addictive than heroin because it's very hard to get off them.
- You do not need to stay on medications for too long. You can stop them if you are doing well.
- Threatening or putting someone in prison will cure them of their addiction. Law enforcement strategies are the best way of decreasing demand for drugs.
- Because you were in a residential program or prison for a long time with no access to drugs, you are no longer addicted. If you relapsed after that, it was your choice and not the disorder.

CHAPTER 7

When Treating OUD Becomes a Challenge

It is Jason's third and most violent suicide attempt. Lacey's oldest daughter comes home to find her dad sitting in his chair slumped over, both wrists slit. She calls the police, and an officer notifies Lacey that they are taking her husband to a nearby psychiatric ward for three days of involuntary observation. Here, Jason is diagnosed with post-traumatic stress disorder (PTSD). He is given a prescription for the antidepressant sertraline and referrals to counseling.

Jason has become obsessed with dying, convinced his days are numbered. Now fifty years old, he is the age at which his father passed. Lacey wonders whether Jason's suicide attempts are a self-fulfilling prophecy. Jason's father, a physically and emotionally abusive alcoholic, haunts his memories. Jason has talked about his traumatic childhood with Lacey, who has on more than one occasion comforted him during a nightmare or flashback. But he is not diagnosed with PTSD until well into his opioid addiction.

From the psych ward, Jason is taken directly to a residential treatment facility for men, his second time in residential rehab. This time, he is forced to stay for forty-five days. The center has a special treatment track for trauma and PTSD. It is a hard-core traditional program with no medications allowed: Jason is required to go cold turkey, even during withdrawal. For this, he will later blame and never forgive Lacey, who does not lift a finger to get him out, despite his ongoing laments. Consumed with anger for having to go through yet another dramatic episode, Lacey is unable to drum up any compassion. She does not visit Jason on the psych ward or at the center. It feels good to let go a little. She feels justified, a small sense of pleasure from finally having a smidgen of control.

Jason comes home from his treatment stint acting a little more like his old self and with some useful behavioral skills. He is vigilant about noting his thoughts about pain and using. "It's just a thought," he reminds himself. He never attends follow-up counseling sessions. Lacey is grateful for his sobriety but leery. She is waiting for the other shoe to drop.

Within a couple of months, after a blowup with Lacey, Jason threatens to leave. Lacey, fed up, tells him to go ahead. To blow off steam and to try and unravel her confused and tangled up thoughts, she heads out the door for a long walk. When she returns about two hours later, she finds Jason passed out on the floor, barely breathing. She calls 911 and rushes to the kitchen cupboard, where she keeps the Narcan. Paramedics arrive, give him oxygen, and transport him to the hospital. When Jason recovers, he voluntarily goes back to rehab. This time he does not go through detox but is started on Suboxone for his opioid use disorder (OUD) and hydroxyzine for anxiety. No one ever talks to him about methadone.

After twenty-eight days, Jason comes home and takes Suboxone for a week or so. Lacey hates that he is taking pills, although she says nothing. It is still something he puts in his mouth, and she is weary of watching him eat pills. He makes no effort to attend the recommended Narcotics Anonymous meetings and does not show up at counseling appointments. His mood has not improved. If anything, he is more obsessed with getting painkillers.

Complex Cases

Medication for OUD can be lifesaving, yet it's not a silver bullet. People with this disorder come from all walks of life and present with assorted complications that challenge even the most skilled practitioners. By the time those with addiction enter treatment, many are sitting atop a sinkhole of problems: hepatitis and other medical issues, social and vocational problems, and housing and financial concerns, as well as psychiatric symptoms. For the best chance at recovery, people with addiction need to address all these issues or they become reasons to use again. For most patients, taking away the drug is not enough. Recovery is not just abstinence but wellness and quality of life and being free from as many problems as possible. True recovery is building strength.

For professionals, policy makers, and family members alike who are not well versed in treatment issues, this chapter serves as a condensed look at some of the more challenging considerations of treating addiction, including working with teenagers, pregnant women, inmates, chronic pain patients, and people with co-occurring mental health issues. Recognizing some of the complications may help you to know when a person would benefit from seeing a mental health or other professional for screening and higher levels of care, as well as what that care might look like. These challenges are not only difficult for the practitioner—they are without a doubt painful for the individual with OUD and are leading causes of relapse.

Mental Illness and Drug Use: The Chicken or the Egg?

It is safe to say that no one comes to treatment because life is great. By the time I see patients, their drugs have stopped working for them, and they've lost jobs and homes, damaged important relationships, and likely acquired medical problems because of their use. Most are also depressed, anxious, or suffering from some other mental health issue. What brings people to treatment is usually the psychological suffering.

How and when they became this way is at first a mystery: depression, anxiety, psychosis, personality problems, and other mental health issues can be the result or the cause of drug use. Nearly half of all people diagnosed with a substance use disorder also have a co-occurring disorder—a mental health issue to accompany addiction—at some point over their life span. The stigma of addiction pales in comparison to that surrounding mental illness. Combine the two—addiction and mental illness—and it adds up to what some in the field call "double trouble." Having both disorders makes everything twice as difficult. These individuals need twice as much treatment and may find it more difficult to respond to treatment and maintain abstinence. Finding and accessing care, a support group, and employment may be harder for them. And caring for someone with co-occurring disorders can be overwhelming, for family members and even health-care providers.

Understanding how addiction and psychiatric symptoms are related is a first step to more effectively helping such individuals. Someone may have a psychiatric disorder and over time develop a substance use disorder, or they may use substances first and over time develop mental health problems. They can find themselves in any of the following scenarios:

- They may have a mental health problem and use drugs to relieve psychiatric symptoms
- Excessive drug use may be one symptoms of their psychiatric disorder
- Drug use may intensify their psychiatric symptoms
- Chronic drug use causes depression or anxiety symptoms to develop
- Drug use can precipitate or trigger a mental health condition

Self-medicating with opioids or other drugs to mask uncomfortable and sometimes undiagnosed mental health symptoms is common. Opioids are such a psychologically powerful medicine that they relieve all sorts of symptoms. They can thwart depression, anxiety, and psychosis all at once. Heroin works amazingly well for quieting the symptoms of

PTSD, including distressing flashbacks. In addition, having a psychiatric disorder often increases the risk that a person will try substances. Jason, for instance, wasn't diagnosed with PTSD until well into his fifties. His first use of opioids at an early age likely had an immediate effect on his PTSD symptoms, which started in childhood. Impulsivity also comes into play. Disorders that make a person more impulsive, such as bipolar disorder or attention-deficit/hyperactivity disorder (ADHD), encourage people to seek out intense experiences, including drug use. Those who use opioids impulsively or to self-medicate and have a genetic vulnerability toward addiction may eventually develop OUD secondary to their psychiatric disorder.

Using drugs to self-medicate unwanted emotions can work temporarily, but eventually it can do the opposite and intensify symptoms of depression or anxiety. For example, someone who starts drinking might at first feel as if alcohol makes living with depression tolerable. As drinking becomes more frequent and heavier, it no longer lifts the depression, which then becomes more pervasive and severe. When this happens, the person who drinks is trapped in cycles of heavier episodes of drinking and deeper, unremitting depression. Opioids can have the same result.

Drugs can also create new moods in a person: A happy-go-lucky individual who starts drinking to excess may develop a newfound melancholy. Like alcohol, opioids are depressants—they slow down the central nervous system, which can, in people vulnerable to depression, create heavy feelings of sadness. Likewise, intoxication with opioids can produce a mellow, worry-free state. Opioid withdrawal produces its own brand of psychiatric syndrome—people who may have felt good on their drug of choice can become agitated and extremely anxious and restless without it, as if they are having an acute anxiety attack.

To add yet another layer of complexity, drug use can also precipitate a mental illness by triggering the expression of certain genes that had until then lain dormant. The classic example is cannabis and schizophrenia. Over and over again, studies have shown that people vulnerable to the mental disorder can trigger it by smoking pot, especially if they start at an early age and smoke large doses of high-potency cannabis. Regardless of the scenario, drug users find themselves in a catch-22: The more they use drugs, the more powerful their depression, anxiety, or other disorder grows, and the more drugs they need to feel better.

Often, people with OUD don't know themselves which came first, the mental health issue or the drug use. They usually can't explain it. It's confusing to them, and they don't understand what's happening to them. It's a chicken-or-egg question. Part of my job is to determine which problem—the mood disorder or the OUD—is driving the other. The answer is important to health-care professionals because it affects how we treat our patients. Whichever course we take, we want to treat both, using all the tools we have: medications, psychotherapy, and, in some cases, an inpatient stay to observe the person drug-free, treat any withdrawal and acute psychiatric symptoms, and then start planning long-term treatment.

What happens when we take away the drugs: a timeline approach

During an evaluation, a first step to solving the puzzle is to ask the patient questions and create a timeline for each problem. *When did you start using substances? Was there a time when you stopped using? When did you start feeling depressed? When did you start to have difficulty sleeping? Were you hyperactive as a child? Did you have trouble going to camp or speaking in front of the class? Did these feelings get worse? When did they get better?* Then, we look at how the timelines overlap.

If symptoms disappeared when the patient was abstinent for a prolonged length of time, because of pregnancy or jail time, for instance, there's a good chance that the substance use caused the mental health disorder. Half of the time, this is the case. People who use drugs develop psychiatric symptoms. A person who binges on cocaine and doesn't sleep for two days might develop psychosis and paranoia, then, after twenty-four hours in the emergency room and a good night's rest, wake up completely lucid. It is clear that the symptoms are a direct effect of the stimulant: Take the cocaine out of the equation for a few weeks and the psychiatric symptoms go away. In the case of opioids, some people will develop feelings of sadness, stop enjoying social events, and lose their appetite and interest in sex. Heroin may make it better for short periods of time, but the depression becomes more severe, hopelessness sets in, and suicide becomes a consideration. Once these individuals are abstinent, however, mood dramatically brightens and sleep, appetite, energy, and sex drive improve in a matter of one to two weeks. Such people do not need treatment for depression—once heroin or illicit painkillers are out of the picture, just monitoring mood may be sufficient. In these cases, treatment of addiction may be easier, as there is only one disorder to deal with, and the prognosis is better.

If the symptoms of depression persist during the first two to four weeks of abstinence, we need to dig a little deeper. We need to assume that depression might have been there before addiction developed, and that it needs to be treated. Treating drug addiction while ignoring a mood disorder or other mental health issue is usually futile, as more often than not it leads to relapse. Delaying treatment of a psychiatric disorder because of the notion that most psychiatric problems were substance induced, a dominant belief among psychiatrists in the past, leads to poor outcomes and unnecessary suffering.

Co-occurring disorders: all ready for treatment but no place to go

In the not-too-distant past, addicted individuals who suffered from an untreated mental health issue were denied addiction treatment. The thinking was that they must first be treated for the mental illness before they could focus on the work of recovery. Success rates for treating people with co-occurring disorders were abominable, and the addiction treatment field saw no other solution. Likewise, mental health professionals declared the opposite: Drugs are usually the cause of mental health issues, so abstinence will unveil any real issues, if they do indeed exist. No psychiatrist wanted to treat patients for an illness they didn't have. Nor did anyone want to give medication to individuals actively using, for fear of what might happen if the drugs interacted in the wrong way. Like fans of two opposing teams, both camps shouted their beliefs from the stands, across a field of potential patients. People with addiction who showed any sign of a co-occurring disorder were left on the sidelines, suffering inadequate treatment.

The problem did not go unrecognized. In the 1980s, the concept of treating co-occurring disorders began to garner a following. Experts tried several approaches. For example, they treated the more "severe" disorder first, or the one that was first diagnosed (the primary disorder). They tried addressing psychiatric problems first, and addiction problems first. Then came the idea of using two different treatment teams to treat both problems at the same time, in parallel, a method known as split treatment.

The most accepted practice now is for one treatment team to recognize and treat both disorders, preferably at the same time. Yet patients run into the same problems that they do with evidence-based treatment for OUD alone: (1) Addiction treatment facilities equipped to treat co-occurring disorders are few and far between. (2) Most traditional programs do not have psychiatrists on staff. (3) Some have consultants visit for one or two hours a week but lack a team of psychologists, therapists, and psychiatrists on board to fully address psychiatric problems. And (4), these settings tend to gloss over patients' symptoms or refer difficult patients elsewhere. It is not that providers argue with the treatment model—it's again a matter of staffing and funding, as well as finding psychiatrists with expertise treating patients with addictions, who are in short supply. As with evidence-based treatments for OUD, patients and family members who are dealing with co-occurring disorders have to know what they are looking for and seek it out.

Treating co-occurring disorders

The new model is integrated treatment: We address the mental health issue at the same time that we treat the addiction. Both are chronic conditions with the possibility of remission and relapse, so that treating one and ignoring the other is a great disservice to the patient. The two disorders are by now tightly woven together. Separating them is arduous. If you only treat the addiction, the patient remains depressed and starts thinking of using to feel better; if you only treat the depression, the patient starts feeling good and decides it can't hurt to use again.

As soon as we know that a patient's psychiatric symptoms are mostly independent of substance use, or existed before the substance use disorder developed, we can address the issue without delay. Treatment comes in the form of behavioral and medical interventions, which might include medications and focused individual and group therapies. The "knowing," however, can take time, at least a few weeks of observation during ongoing abstinence. By then, patients stabilizing on naltrexone, buprenorphine, or methadone have gone through acute and most of the protracted withdrawal. What appeared to be a psychiatric symptom may have disappeared by then. It is common for depressed mood, chronic fatigue, anxiety, and suicidal ideation to be replaced with abundant energy, optimism, and a newly found interest in hobbies. For instance, someone who had periods of extreme irritability, euphoric moods, and even psychotic states and was diagnosed with bipolar disorder may become levelheaded, with stable, normal mood. But that isn't the end of treatment: Should the symptoms of a disorder persist, or get worse despite abstinence from drugs, we are wise to treat it aggressively. Wait too long and the person will relapse. Any untreated psychiatric disorder makes recovery that much harder.

In an ideal world, we would wait through one or two months of abstinence before calling a psychiatric disorder preexisting. But addiction and mental illness is not an ideal world. Prescribed medications might take one or two weeks to kick in. So, even though we are observing, evaluating, and assessing the patient, we face a four- to six-week impasse when psychiatric treatment is at a standstill and the patient is at an ever-increasing risk of relapsing. Close monitoring and intensive therapeutic support are essential during this time.

When two become one

Patients are tempted to lend more importance to one disorder than the other, but I agree with the approach that gives each equal weight and treats such people as having one disorder—"opioid use and depressive disorder," for instance—rather than a primary versus a secondary disorder. This is helpful for the patients as well, who see that the disorders are heavily intertwined and that staying away from problematic drugs helps recovery from the psychiatric disorder and that taking psychiatric medications helps recovery from the addiction. Both disorders can produce irrational thinking and a failure to consider consequences, or impair the ability to care for oneself, which can lead to errors in judgment.

The behavioral therapies we use address both (or multiple) disorders in one fell swoop: cognitive behavioral therapy and relapse prevention strategies, for instance, work through ambivalence about medication treatment and focus on activities and skills that help patients navigate toward recovery from both disorders, regardless of which disorder patients consider to be "primary." Patients also learn much-needed coping skills for high-risk situations, such as what to do when attending a wedding where drugs and using buddies are present, as well as for self-monitoring of cravings and defeatist thought patterns characteristic of a depressive disorder. People in recovery can easily talk themselves into using again without ever saying a word out loud. Therapy helps those in recovery to reroute a negative train of thought to something more useful to protect themselves against relapse. We show them how to modify their lifestyles so that self-care and relationships get more of their attention: Even simple acts, such as making haircut and doctor appointments, and of course being more present with loved ones, can help them stay on track. When the right hand knows what the left hand is doing, treatment success rates for both disorders are quite good.

The approach is straightforward and works when followed. Dr. Roger Weiss, a Harvard addiction psychiatrist, coined a phrase that I really like. He talks about a "central recovery rule," which can be discussed with a therapist at every opportunity and used by the person in recovery as a kind of mantra, repeated in particular when they struggle: "Don't drink, don't use drugs, and take your medications as prescribed no matter what."

Pregnancy and Opioids

There is a myth that women who have misused drugs cannot by definition be good mothers. But this is far from the truth. I've seen many women become abstinent when they find out they are pregnant, start taking care of themselves, and transfer this care to their newborn. They are devoted moms and willing to take professional advice to improve their parenting. For many women, pregnancy is a reason to get off opioids, and the thought of not being able to care for their child fills them with an intense desire to seek help. Yet this is a difficult step to take. Aware of being judged, addicted pregnant women absorb the shame and stigma—both of which are major deterrents to getting good treatment and seeking help. Yet with support, encouragement, and reassurance, along with good medical care, the mother-to-be can have a comfortable, healthy pregnancy, deliver a healthy baby, and be a wonderful new mom.

Take her to see a doctor

Testing of pregnant women for alcohol or drug use is not universal. I recommend that all pregnant women be screened for substances, with the caveat that doctors remain friendly, supportive, and nonjudgmental regardless of the outcome. A big problem is that women who are using substances may fear the legal consequences and choose to neglect pregnancy and newborn care rather than submit to a drug test. In some states, doctors may be mandated to report mothers with substance use problems to child services agencies, while other states offer specialized treatment programs for pregnant women. Pregnant women struggling with addiction should seek legal or trusted professional advice about the state laws with regard to substance use and pregnancy to make an informed choice about treatment for substance use disorder. But identifying and treating a substance use disorder as early as possible is in everyone's best interests.

Like all pregnant women, those with OUD need good obstetric care, preferably from a doctor who has experience with high-risk pregnancies or at least is friendly toward women who use substances. Ideally, the woman would visit the doctor as soon as possible, tell the obstetrician of her addiction, and get regular checkups so the pregnancy is monitored. The sooner she starts to see a doctor, the better.

Seek treatment for OUD

For the best outcome, pregnant women with OUD need to stop using their drug of choice. The risk of overdose is too great. If the mother-to-be takes too much of an opioid, she might pass out, her breathing may slow down or stop, and she could die or have a miscarriage or a stillbirth. Pregnant women who abuse opioids are also in a very unstable physical state, with periods of opioid intoxication and withdrawal. Heroin and painkillers cross the placenta and get to the fetus. This is not a good environment for fetal development and growth and may lead to premature and complicated labor, which can sicken the newborn.

Untreated addiction in pregnant women has also been linked to high-risk behaviors such as prostitution and crime, which can create a cascade of problems: sexually transmitted infections, violence, legal troubles, and incarceration. A mother-to-be needs proper treatment and support, as early in the pregnancy as possible. Loving family members and friends can help to keep trouble at arm's length by encouraging her to seek help for her addiction and get good medical care.

Medication-assisted treatment is recommended

Some women who become pregnant while using opioids want to stop using opioids on their own, in secrecy, but this is very risky. Studies have shown that 8 out of 10 pregnant women return to drug use within a month after detoxing on their own and are at greater risk of overdose. In addition, going through opioid withdrawal with no medical support, she and the fetus will experience complete withdrawal, which can result in significant risks to the pregnancy and the fetus.

Offering medication-assisted treatment during pregnancy is the recommended best practice for the care of pregnant women with OUD. Most doctors treat OUD in pregnant women with either methadone or buprenorphine. These medications stop withdrawal, reduce cravings, and prevent further use of illicit opioids. Under medical supervision, methadone or buprenorphine can reduce the risk of complications in pregnancy and labor. These medications are generally safe for the developing fetus and give the mother-to-be a chance to focus on prenatal care and her addiction treatment and recovery goals. As of yet, naltrexone is not recommended for use in pregnancy, mostly because there is very little experience with it. However, initial experience with naltrexone implants in Australia supports its safety and effectiveness for pregnancy and the newborn.

Treatment of pregnant women with OUD involves taking medications in prescribed doses during pregnancy and after the baby is born. The counseling component helps women avoid and cope with situations that might lead to relapse and supports them through supports them through the process of tackling their addiction. Treatment with methadone is available only in specialized OTP clinics. Buprenorphine may be available from an OTP or a primary care physician or obstetrician who received special training to prescribe buprenorphine.

Methadone used to be the gold standard for treating pregnant women, but this is slowly changing as we gain research and clinical experience with buprenorphine. If a woman wishes to be treated with buprenorphine, providers should offer it over methadone. The preferred formulation of buprenorphine for use in pregnancy is a buprenorphine-only tablet. If, however, she became pregnant while being treated for OUD with methadone, she should be encouraged to remain on methadone. Some pregnant women may need to increase their dose of medicine, or to take it twice per day as they grow in the third trimester, to account for the presence of the growing fetus. They can go back to the lower dose after delivery.

Methadone and buprenorphine cross the placenta and make it to the fetus. Both of these medications carry some risks to the fetus, including a smaller birth weight, though most children eventually catch up in growth and develop normally. These risks are much milder as compared to risks from the use of heroin or other opioids, which also cross over to the fetus.

Decisions about the best course of addiction treatment are best made by each mother-to-be, with the help of doctors and providers who specialize in treating pregnant women. A thorough discussion of the risks and benefits of all treatment decisions should take place, and the doctor should evaluate which treatment setting and medication guarantee the best outcome. Facilities that specialize in treating pregnant women and their families can be found by calling your state's substance abuse services agency. Encourage the mother-to-be to begin treatment for OUD and support her during treatment, through labor, and afterward.

When MAT Is Not an Option

If a pregnant woman prefers to be completely drug-free, or the state mandates complete detoxification, then medication-assisted treatment (MAT), will not be an option. If she does want to receive MAT but it's not available, then consider a medically supervised withdrawal. In this case, a doctor experienced in treating prenatal addiction should supervise care, with the informed consent of the woman. If she needs to come off opioids, the best time is during the second trimester, when the pregnancy is more stable. Undergoing opioid withdrawal during the first trimester may cause miscarriage, and during the last trimester may cause premature labor.

Preparing for delivery

Delivery for pregnant women with OUD is usually no different than any other delivery, but it does require some additional preparation. First and foremost, it is not an option for the woman to hide the fact that she is taking OUD medication therapy. Many women need a pain management plan for childbirth. The usual doses of methadone or buprenorphine will not treat her pain adequately. The mother-to-be should discuss pain control options with her physician during her prenatal care. She must also let the doctors at the hospital know that she is taking methadone or buprenorphine, so they give her medication that will be helpful and not cause problems. Ideally, the doctor and hospital would have experience working with such women during labor and delivery. At a minimum, they need to be accepting and nonjudgmental. That a patient chooses to be in treatment and is taking responsibility for the well-being of her baby and herself deserves support from the medical community.

The mother-to-be also needs to select a doctor for the baby (a pediatrician or family physician) and meet before delivery to talk about the care of her baby. It is important that this doctor is aware that the mother has been taking methadone or buprenorphine during the pregnancy, and that the baby may need additional monitoring or treatment after delivery. A pediatrician will check the baby after birth and decide whether any medications are needed to help the baby during withdrawal. The baby may need to stay in the hospital for a few days or weeks while taking the medication, until they're completely well. Friends and family members can play a large role in encouraging the mother to have these discussions with her doctors as far in advance as possible.

Women are often afraid their babies will be taken away

Many babies and mothers get tested for alcohol and other drugs at delivery. A positive drug test, even if it's the result of prescribed medications, may mean that social workers or a child protection agency will want to talk with the mother and her family. A child services worker may come to the mother's home to see how safe the environment is for her baby, so it is important to prepare for that. In most cases, child protective services wants to keep the family together, and this is especially true if the new mother is actively involved in treatment. Staying on the medication improves chances that she will be able to care for the baby. Be aware of your state's laws and practices regarding drug tests and newborns, and ensure that the mother-to-be is aware of the possible visits from child protective services. The thought of having a child taken away is frightening, to say the least. Reassuring the recovering mom and encouraging her to continue treatment and her new, healthy lifestyle has a calming effect.

The newborn's health

Babies born to women who are addicted to heroin or prescription opioids have been exposed to a similar amount of opioids as the mother. When the baby is born, the supply of opioids is suddenly "cut off," and the baby can have temporary withdrawal or abstinence symptoms called neonatal abstinence syndrome (NAS). Because both methadone and buprenorphine are also opioids, NAS can also occur in babies whose mothers are on methadone or buprenorphine. It does not mean that the baby is born addicted to opioids; it only means that the baby will be born with some physical distress due to exposure to the medications, which can be medically managed. NAS is a treatable condition with a full recovery in all newborns as long as the newborn has no other medical problems.

Every baby shows withdrawal differently. Some will have mild symptoms and others will not show any signs. Symptoms usually occur on the second or third day after birth and can include shaking and tremors, poor feeding or sucking, incessant crying, fever, vomiting, and sleep problems. Doctors may administer medications to ease these symptoms and may keep the baby in the hospital for a few extra days. Some babies may have discomfort related to withdrawal in the very short term, but in the long term, babies with NAS grow as they would normally. NAS causes no known lasting physical or intellectual problems in the baby. What happens to babies after birth has a much larger impact on their development. Being raised by a mother who is well and in recovery from opioid addiction is a big plus.

NAS can be diminished by "rooming in," or being near the mother, breastfeeding, swaddling, and skin-to-skin contact, such as holding baby bare chest to bare chest. Breastfeeding is often encouraged for women who are taking methadone or buprenorphine. Only minuscule amounts of medication get into the breast milk, and this has been shown to help lessen the symptoms of NAS. However, breastfeeding is not safe for women with HIV who are taking certain medicines or who have relapsed and are actively using drugs.

The weeks and months after delivery

Medication and therapy should continue after delivery: The mom needs tender loving care and support. Ensuring she has help in learning how to be a mom and has someone available to take care of any other children for periods of time goes a long way. The weeks and months after a baby is born can be a stressful time for women in general, and even more so for those in recovery. The new mother should be sure to continue substance use disorder treatment, including staying on medication and attending parenting support programs and counseling or relapse prevention programs. This is not a time to stop medications or therapy. The longer people remain on the medication, the better the chance that they will avoid relapse. The dose of the medication may need to be adjusted after the delivery.

The weight of the world

The stigma around addiction and pregnant women is compounded: There is stigma with addiction. There is stigma with addiction in women. And there is even more stigma with addiction in pregnant woman. If she has a mental health issue as well, she is carrying not only a child but the weight of the world on her shoulders. Pregnant women with OUD need support and meaningful advice, not judgment. Helping her find a suitable obstetrician is a great start. From there, she will need ongoing reassurance and support from friends and family, who could offer to go with her to prenatal appointments and encourage her to eat nutritious foods and practice relaxation and stress-relieving techniques. Family members should be open to participating in family therapy, if available.

Adolescents, Teenagers, and Young Adults

Most teenagers will at least experiment with alcohol and other drugs at some point. In some respects, it is a rite of passage, a common denominator of all generations. Curiosity, peer pressure, anxiety, or rebelliousness likely play a role in the decision as well. Many will decide that drugs are not for them and simply return to the activities of their youth, unfazed by what their partying peers think of them. Others will dabble for a bit, drink too much beer on occasion, smoke cannabis once in a while, but not take any of it too seriously. Still others will go full throttle and make drug use the center of their teenage existence, yet easily and gladly walk away from the world of drugs as if it never really mattered within the space of ten years. A small fraction of the tens of thousands of adolescents out there experimenting with drugs, however, will start showing signs of addiction before age twenty. The problem is identifying which teens are likely to do so.

We do not have a blood test to identify high-risk adolescents. We have to rely on the traditional tool of a clinical interview. Children who grow up exposed to neglect or abuse, and those with a family history of addiction or psychiatric disorders, are at higher risk for developing substance use disorders. Adolescents with a history of psychological problems or psychiatric disorders as a child, especially if those remain undiagnosed and untreated, will also be at high risk of developing addiction. Growing up in neighborhoods where violence and drugs are often present, with peers who use drugs, and with limited opportunities for non-drug-related social or recreational activities can contribute to the genetic risks and result in addiction in a teenager.

Nothing is simple or straightforward about diagnosing a teenager with substance use disorder. Distinguishing between the follies of youth and a substance use disorder is not clear-cut, especially because many adolescents will neither see nor accept that they have lost the ability to control their substance use. They will not ask for help until it is very late. Others around them need to be the ones to identify it as a problem: parents, teachers, pediatricians, and friends. Routine medical and psychological visits provide opportunity for asking adolescents about substance use.

If physicians seem genuinely interested and inquire in an accepting and nonjudgmental manner, teenagers are generally open and talk about their experiences with substances, more so if they can be assured of confidentiality and no immediate negative consequences.

Identifying an adolescent with problematic drug use early on can minimize the toxic effects of substances on the vulnerable and developing brain. Intervening early on can be much more effective in reversing pathological brain changes and preventing further physical and psychological harm that comes with the lifestyle of a regular drug user. Disrupting further exposure to substances is a priority at this stage.

Treating teens

Identifying adolescents who have developed drug use disorder is difficult at best, but treating them is a bit of a mystery. Adolescents may not see the value of treatment and may not have not developed their language and thinking fully enough to express themselves, be introspective, and engage in psychological treatment. They therefore may require different treatment techniques than those developed for adults.

Treatment should target the whole person, not just the problematic drug use, which for adolescents covers a wide swath of developmental skills. As young people, they are already tasked with a monumental job: learning how to navigate the world of people, emotions, social pressures, difficult decisions, and conflict. They don't have everything figured out, and substance use can cloud this process even more. When adolescents take drugs, they are at the same time feeling grown-up and actually stalling their development: Using drugs hinders the learning of some developmental skills; the drug eases social anxiety or masks hurtful feelings, negating the need for introspection and more mature responses.

Identifying and addressing risk factors and external circumstances that may contribute to teens' ongoing drug use is essential to successful treatment. Helping adolescents develop and improve personal and social skills improves treatment outcomes. Educating them about what is required for a healthy sex life, minimizing intimate violence, and preventing sexually transmitted diseases are also important factors of treatment. Because adolescents' lives involve school, hobbies, sports, and peer groups, treatment should support a drug-free life in all of those arenas. Encouraging family members to support the treatment plan and educate and guide their loved one through difficult times goes a long way toward keeping young people who use opioids sober.

Treatment for teens often involves a residential stay as the first step. They spend a month or more in an addiction rehabilitation facility where they have a chance to be drug-free and recover physically. A team of providers is usually on board to evaluate and begin treating co-occurring psychiatric disorders, such as depression or anxiety. Young people in treatment learn about the effects of drugs on the body and mind, how to recognize triggers for relapse, and how to avoid them by using newly learned skills. They can also learn and practice new personal and social skills. Most programs will also introduce teens to the Twelve Step approach to recovery and set a plan at discharge to use their new skills to help them stay sober once they get home.

Still, as yet there is no surefire technique. At fifteen or sixteen, teenagers are told they cannot use drugs, not even legal drugs, ever, for the rest of their lives. Ambivalence is high posttreatment, and such concepts don't always take hold. Youths are hard to treat. We don't fully understand how to treat them—should treatment be short-term, lifelong, or somewhere in between? In truth, we need more research.

OUD medication and teenagers

The use of medication to treat teenagers with OUD remains controversial. Long-term studies of teens treated with medications are nonexistent, and it is difficult to reconcile the idea that a young person may need lifelong treatment with medication. Traditional treatment involved methadone maintenance. Very few methadone programs treated sixteen- and seventeen-year-olds. Most programs required, and still require, patients to be a minimum of eighteen years old. Buprenorphine is FDA approved for patients aged sixteen and over and is an option for a large number of adolescents with OUD. However, even fewer teens are offered treatment with medications than adults.

Similar to adults, the longer that adolescent patients are maintained on buprenorphine, the better the outcome. The evidence is limited but suggests that most patients should be encouraged to remain on buprenorphine in the long term, especially if they are doing well. Some providers prefer that adolescents' treatment with buprenorphine be time limited to one to two years of sobriety, even though no data suggest that this is a good strategy.

The major challenge is to get teens to keep taking their medication. Adolescents are less likely to comply over the long term than adults. The additional challenge is that they may not be responsible enough to hold their supply of buprenorphine. The controlled substance can be diverted, misused, or simply lost, like a set of car keys. We need innovative strategies to help teens adhere to their medications, perhaps strategies that harness the power of social media and gamification.

One of the best strategies is to involve parents in treatment. Parents can securely store the medication and allot their child only a daily dose. Even better, parents can directly supervise each time the medication is taken. It is best to do it first thing in the morning, when the teen may still be in bed. When just waking up, or before they get busy, adolescents are more likely to put the tablet or the film in their mouth. After a few minutes of sitting at the bedside, a parent is reassured that the medication has been absorbed and this day their child will be protected against relapse and overdose. This ritual has to be repeated day after day, but most parents, who understand its importance, are happy to do it. Teens grow to like it as well, especially if it becomes part of a warm, daily greeting that puts a positive spin on the day ahead. The mother of one of my patients lies down with her daughter after giving her the medication. The two are reassured and connected through the gesture. It is as much for the mom as it is for the child. The alternative to a daily supervised dose of buprenorphine may be a long-acting buprenorphine injection.

Naltrexone, by tablet or injection, is not approved for use in children younger than eighteen because we know little about its safety and effectiveness in this population. The few centers that do offer XR-naltrexone to young adults experience mostly positive results. Long-acting naltrexone is a particular favorite of parents as a treatment option for their children. Parents like the assurance that the injection offers—it beats praying every time your children leave the house that they don't score opioids somewhere and die of an overdose. With XR-naltrexone, parents can watch their children take the monthly dose and know that, if they do use, the drug effects will be blocked. They will not get high. They will not overdose. And they will not die. It is not the easy way out. It is the sane, logical way. Naltrexone may soon be available as an implant lasting several months and offering greater reassurance.

Most adolescents (like many adults) do not like the idea of taking medication indefinitely. They tend to like the idea of using buprenorphine in the long term even less than naltrexone, because they will still be on opioids. We are not sure how long patients need to stay on naltrexone, but we do know that it may need to be longer than one or two years. In practice, it is difficult to keep teens on the injection for more than eighteen to twenty-four months. They grow weary of taking the medication, even if they are doing well. But during this period of time in the life of an adolescent, when brain and psychological development is at a pinnacle, OUD medication is invaluable. It allows for normal psychological development to continue, whereas heroin and other drugs interfere with development. Little in life matters when you are in the grip of addiction. At this point, we do not know whether chronic exposure to medication, be it an agonist or antagonist, alters neurological pathways or the normal development of higher cortical functions. As always, taking medication has to be weighed against the risk of relapse and death.

Prevention: A vaccine for addiction?

The other quandary is how to keep all adolescents, whether they're just out to have fun or needing a fix, safe from deadly overdoses. We know that the opioids available today are insanely potent. If drugs are seen as a rite of passage, and the drugs available today are deadly, an entire generation is being not only duped but possibly fatally betrayed by their own culture. Adolescents are not always mature enough to understand the potential consequences of taking drugs. Most young people, for instance, do not overdose intentionally. Rarely is overdose connected to suicide in youths. It's almost always an accident—a bad combination of opioids, sedatives, and alcohol, or unwittingly taking street drugs fortified with fentanyl or some other unexpected substance. They're just kids—many of them with loving and beaming personalities—who make a poor choice in the wrong place at the wrong time.

All providers should alert parents who know or suspect that their child is taking opioids to seek training on overdose recognition and prevention. These parents should keep one or more doses of naloxone on hand. It is very unsettling to have to be prepared for a child's overdose, but the idea of being helpless in this situation is even more horrifying. Grassroots organizations, run by parents whose kids have died of opioid overdoses, offer free trainings on how to deliver naloxone to an overdose victim. Countless times, because families are able to act in time, overdoses are prevented.

Traditional, evidence-based methods of prevention that are proving successful, especially those targeted at high-risk youths, include programs that bolster psychological development and teach basic living skills that went unlearned during years of heavy using. However, untargeted prevention, such as public service announcements and police officers visiting schools, is not demonstrably effective.

I once again advocate for the health-care system to get more involved. During annual exams, when pediatricians make a point to discuss sexual health, they could just as easily broach the subject of drug use and even take a confidential urine toxicology test. If necessary, they could conduct a brief intervention. If framed as a way to address overall health, not as a punitive measure, these conversations could greatly increase awareness. Being watched, or monitored, in this way sends the message to youth that adults care what happens to them and that they are accountable for their health.

Criminal Justice System

Every year, about one third of illicit opioid users find themselves behind cell doors, locked up in a correctional facility for one crime or another. About one quarter of all inmates have OUD. Most often, their offense is nonviolent and secondary to having an addiction, such as drug possession or sale, or petty theft. Most of them would not be committing crimes were it not for their addiction. Having such a large number of individuals with OUD in a controlled environment is a great opportunity to offer treatment, which not only benefits the health of an inmate but decreases the spread of infectious diseases, addresses risk factors for reoffending, and greatly benefits public health and security. Yet a great majority of incarcerated individuals with OUD are left untreated. Within three months of release, three quarters of them will relapse to heroin use, even after being referred to treatment in the community. Many will continue their criminal activities. Tragically, many others will overdose when they relapse and never have an opportunity to benefit from treatment.

Upon entry, most new inmates with OUD must go through a forced detoxification. Only a handful of jails and prisons offer medication to ease withdrawal symptoms. Detoxification followed by abstinence is the intended outcome for most prisoners, at least while within prison walls, in most facilities. When a prison offers a drug treatment program, it is usually abstinence based. Rarely is a program based on the medical model. Some US prisons offer methadone. In facilities that offer methadone maintenance, about half restrict the treatment to pregnant women and inmates with chronic pain; even when an inmate comes in on methadone, they may not have the option to continue with it. This practice is very different from that of most other developed countries, where methadone or buprenorphine treatment is widely available in prisons. Even countries that only recently introduced methadone, such as Iran, are now offering it in prisons because the benefits are hard to argue with.

This is yet another situation where a poor understanding of OUD has grave consequences. OUD is a chronic disorder that is unlikely to be "cured" by forced abstinence during incarceration, and psychosocial treatments are rarely sufficient. If left untreated, drug cravings and use will recur, usually as soon as the person becomes exposed to drug triggers and gains access to drugs. Forced abstinence is not treatment. Relapse should be expected on discharge, and referral to an outpatient program, even if that program offers medications, is not enough.

Treatment in prison should be the same as the treatment offered to the general population, similar to treatment offered for other medical conditions. Treatment with medication should be the mainstay. Individuals stabilized on medication are more likely to have fewer psychological symptoms and take advantage of psychosocial interventions and all the other rehabilitative programs offered in prison. Additional psychosocial programs and self-help groups may also be offered. On discharge, individuals stabilized on medication are not only less likely to immediately relapse and overdose, they are also more likely to continue with treatment in the community, adhering to the medication, and attending programs and self-help groups.

If we offer treatment with medication to all inmates with OUD, they are much less likely to be reincarcerated. Medication, backed by some newly learned living skills and behavioral therapies, gives them at least a fighting chance when confronted with difficult circumstances upon reentry, including being surrounded by drug use, rejection from family and employers, and feelings of hopelessness. Offering medication in prison but especially before release, along with some degree of aftercare, not only saves but improves lives and reinforces the separation between addiction and the criminal justice system.

Why referral to treatment after prison is not enough

Treatment with medications is well proven to improve health and reduce recidivism, but many newly released inmates are reluctant to take the medications. Some fear they will become addicted to methadone or buprenorphine, which might reflect attitudes expressed toward medications by treatment providers in prison. Ex-inmates also fear that if reincarcerated, they will have to go through yet another traumatic opioid withdrawal from buprenorphine or methadone. In such cases, treatment with naltrexone may be a preferred option. Individuals who were recently involved in the criminal justice system and were treated with XR-naltrexone are much more likely to remain abstinent and engaged in treatment than those referred to a traditional treatment program. The traditional belief that abstinence is the only real recovery also prevails. Using medication feels like a step backward, especially for those who stay years in prison drug-free. However, its benefits are hard to argue with.

Furthermore, when former prisoners are interested in starting treatment with medication, they may have difficulty finding services, have to wait too long to get medication, or may not have the resources needed to cover the cost of treatment. If free treatment services were available for this population on release, many would avoid reincarceration, which is much more costly.

Chronic Pain and OUD

We know that chronic pain and chronic opioid use are not synonymous, but a percentage of people who are prescribed opioids for chronic pain have OUD, and most of them are undiagnosed and untreated. In these individuals, OUD developed directly as a result of treatment with opioid painkillers. We cannot eliminate painkillers. We cannot deny relief to patients in palliative care or hospice, for instance, where risk of addiction is not an issue and treatment focuses on maximizing pain relief. Nor can we ignore the 11 percent of Americans who suffer from chronic pain. We cannot stop prescribing painkillers for recovery after surgery or a serious acute injury condition. Nor can we turn a blind eye to the fact that a simple prescription can in a few months' time lead to heroin and fentanyl use and eventually destroy an entire family. How do we address pain and prevent addiction at the same time?

In 2016, twenty years after the opioid prescription frenzy began, the Centers for Disease Control and Prevention (CDC) came out with guidelines for prescribing opioids to patients with chronic pain that high-light addiction as a major consideration. Compared to earlier guidelines, the CDC recommends lower dosages, refers to *all* patients (except those in palliative care and hospice) as being at "high risk" for OUD, and offers more specific recommendations for how to know when the risks outweigh the benefits. It was a long-awaited step in the right direction.

Treating chronic pain is complex. It is true that if the doctor can identify the cause, the patient has severe chronic pain that is responding to opioids, and there's an 80 percent chance that the patient will not acquire an addiction, then taking opioids might seem like a good gamble.

This gamble comes with a litany of assumptions, namely that doctors will be able to detect when someone starts becoming addicted and will do something to stop it.

When it comes to the chronic pain conundrum, two very major considerations are almost always overlooked: First, the body naturally develops a tolerance to opioids. Sooner or later, the painkillers will stop working. Nonaddicted pain patients may not crave more opioids, but will experience pain that can now only be relieved with more opioids. Second, painkillers, in time, will not only stop working but also cause increased pain in some patients. In these cases, opioids have sensitized the body, and patients experience more severe pain. These patients find relief only when taken off painkillers.

A range of nonopioid medications and behavioral strategies are available that could be helpful for some people. And, in the midst of our public health emergency, the call to develop nonaddictive painkillers more potent than Tylenol is loud and clear. But in the end, we have to set the expectation that some people will have to live with some pain. The assumption that everyone should have 100 percent of their pain taken away is unrealistic—and quite recent. Up until the 1980s, most Americans outside of a hospital setting took aspirin or Tylenol for pain relief. Eliminating 100 percent of pain in all patients will likely not be possible, as it is not possible to cure many illnesses that cause pain. Making 100 percent pain relief a priority carries too big a risk for the population at large, especially if we think that opioids are the solution. Opioid painkillers are powerful and potentially dangerous medicines, hence they are not available over the counter.

These reasons alone are enough to advocate for pulling back on prescribing opioids to patients who don't show any real evidence of pain relief and turning instead to less potent but safer pain relievers and nonmedication methods, such as massage, yoga, acupuncture, and meditation. Beyond that, medical professionals should follow the selective prescribing practices outlined in the 2016 CDC guidelines, which advocate for only prescribing very low doses for short periods of time. If the medication doesn't relieve pain, doctors should not prescribe more but find something else that does help. How to enforce this approach is another story, but accepting that we have to do something to stop unnecessary initiations to opioids is important if we are at all serious about curtailing the opioid epidemic's accelerating growth.

Another issue is that when doctors stop prescribing opioids, the 20 percent of patients who are dependent will eventually turn to street drugs. This is a clear and unintended consequence, yet we know that, without intervention, it will happen sooner or later for all but a few. Once those patients have been exposed to opioids long enough to become physically dependent, efforts must focus on harm reduction and treatment. Our best hope is preventing exposure to new initiates by trying other, more holistic methods of pain relief first or dispensing more innocent drugs, such as aspirin or ibuprofen, for pain whenever possible.

Treating OUD patients who have chronic pain

Half of all patients being treated for OUD experience pain, and those in recovery from OUD may at some point experience acute or chronic pain worthy of a shot of morphine. If treating chronic pain in otherwise healthy people is complex, it is an even thornier problem for doctors facing patients who are being treated for opioid addiction while complaining of pain. Doctors and patients find themselves in a difficult situation. The stigma of both conditions leads some providers to question the legitimacy of complaints of pain or even reject them outright. In acute situations, providers may not offer treatment that would be offered to patients without addiction. Patients, likewise are reluctant to volunteer information about their OUD because they fear prejudice and mistreatment.

Patients treated with methadone or buprenorphine who experience pain should be offered additional, and highly supervised, pain treatment. Prescribers should work in concert with the patient's addiction provider. Not addressing pain puts patients in stress and at risk of relapse. Even though methadone and buprenorphine are pain relievers, the doses and dosing frequency used for addiction are not sufficient to provide pain relief. First, the patient is usually tolerant to the maintenance doses. The body adapts and the pain threshold goes up. Patients maintained on methadone and buprenorphine feel pain the same as do other people who are not treated with these medications. Second, these medications produce pain relief for only a few hours after the dose, as opposed to the antiwithdrawal effect, which lasts all day.

In patients maintained on methadone who require treatment for acute pain, the maintenance dose should be continued and additional pain medications offered, but higher and more frequent doses may be needed. In the case of chronic pain, a higher dose of methadone may be necessary, preferably given two or three times per day, if possible.

Less is known about treatment of pain in patients treated with buprenorphine. But as with methadone, the maintenance dose of buprenorphine is continued and additional pain medicine is added. Alternatively, the buprenorphine dose can be increased, with a dose given every four to six hours. And in yet another scenario, buprenorphine can be stopped, and traditional opioid painkillers used as long as the pain is severe. In this case, once the patient no longer needs treatment for pain, the buprenorphine is reintroduced.

It is important that patients discuss the fact they are being treated with OUD medications before scheduled surgery, so that the best approach can be planned. In general, stopping medications days before a planned surgery is ill-advised. The patient may become destabilized and have unnecessary anxiety and even cravings, putting them at risk of relapse. Stopping buprenorphine or methadone one day before a scheduled surgery is usually sufficient. Some addiction experts even suggest that the daily dose of buprenorphine should not be stopped, as additional pain can be managed using more potent opioids that are available in the hospital setting.

Pain management in patients treated with naltrexone is more complex. Naltrexone is a very effective blocker of opioids, and standard doses will not get onto receptors and will have no effect on pain. The blockade from naltrexone tablets lasts for two to three days after the last dose and five to six weeks after the last naltrexone injection. However, this blockade can be overcome using very high doses of potent opioids. Doses ten to twenty times higher than the standard dose may be needed to "overcome" the blockade.

Patients treated with naltrexone are wise to wear a medical bracelet or carry a naltrexone card in their wallet. In case of an emergency, such as a car accident, an anesthesiologist can administer high enough doses of opioids to provide needed pain relief, but it needs to be done under careful observation to monitor breathing. Patients can also be anesthetized without using opioids.

For acute pain that does not require surgery, patients who are blocked with naltrexone can be treated with nonopioid medications, such as anti-inflammatory agents, muscle relaxants, anticonvulsants, or others. Nonmedication strategies can also be used, such as local nerve blockers and anesthetic injections under the skin. If surgery is required but can be postponed, it is best to schedule it for after the effect of naltrexone is expected to wear off. Even though many patients and providers are worried about the problem with pain management in patients on naltrexone, in practice, problems related to pain are very rare.

PART 3

A Brief Guide for Families

CHAPTER 8

How to Encourage Your Loved One to Get Help—and How to Help Yourself

Samantha comes home from the pharmacy and plops the weightless brown paper bag on the kitchen counter, as she has done a half dozen times before. It contains a box of needles—syringes her son Eric, now twenty-four years old, is expecting. As soon as he hears the door slam shut, he glides down the stairs into the kitchen, grabs the bag, thanks his mom, and heads out to Jefferson Avenue to get a fix. Samantha makes sure the unused needles and her son are gone before her husband, Tom, comes home from work. Tom knows she is supplying their son with opioid paraphernalia, but he only begrudgingly approves. So, as far as Samantha is concerned, the less he sees, the better.

Samantha's sister doesn't approve at all. She calls it enabling. Samantha's parents think she is crazy and that she should call the police when Eric comes home high. Only "tough love" will get Eric to stop. The pharmacist has started rolling his eyes slightly in a show of contempt when Samantha asks for more needles. But she turns a blind eye to the criticism. It is not that she approves of Eric's use. It's just that she'd rather see him graduate from college someday and maybe even walk down the aisle than be "right." She wants her son. Her real son. But she will take him here on earth as he is, alive and shooting up heroin, rather than reject him or watch him waste away from a drug-related infection caused by something as preventable as dirty needles.

Samantha knows that Eric is going to use whether she approves or not. She's already tried every trick in the book to get him to stop, all to no avail. She could kick him out of the house, but that won't help her cause. Samantha knows that opioid use disorder (OUD) is the most lethal of substance use and psychiatric disorders. Every time Eric decides to use an opioid, there's a small chance he'll die, from an overdose or infection, in an accident, or by dealing with the wrong people in the wrong neighborhood. She's well aware that opioid use comes with some irreversible consequences. So, she does what she can to keep him alive.

Supplying him with clean needles means keeping him from contracting hepatitis C, HIV, or some other dangerous skin or vein infection— helping him to cheat death or a lifelong illness, at least in one small way. But she does more than buy needles. Samantha has provided Eric with the location of the nearest opioid harm reduction center, where he can learn which drugs not to mix and how to use safely, as well as get his street drugs tested before injecting them so he knows he's not taking enough to knock out an elephant. She also stocks her home with items she'll need if Eric goes through withdrawal or overdose—over-the-counter medications and naloxone, the opioid overdose antidote. She does all this to keep her son alive in preparation for the inevitable—that point in time when he is ready to seek help.

So, in spite of the criticism from others, Samantha doesn't waver. She goes to the pharmacy and buys the hypodermic needles. Religiously. Every month.

Samantha, at the advice of a counselor, is employing two strategies—harm reduction and a practice known as motivational interviewing—to help get Eric to *want* to seek treatment. These strategies are rooted in love and forgiveness but based on foresight and evidence. They are counterintuitive, so doing them can feel confusing. Committing to them is not always easy, but it is doable. Employing them requires strength, courage, diligence, and a certain level of trust and compassion. Not everyone has these traits—especially those of you who have been dealing with someone with OUD for a long time. Regardless of how much compassion you have for the person with OUD, I encourage you to read through this chapter. Its approach is based on the work of doctors William R. Miller, Stephen Rollnick, Robert J. Meyers, and Jane Ellen Smith, among others, and has been widely adopted. At some point, you might find the skills outlined here to be useful.

We covered harm reduction strategies used by social workers in chapter 3, pages 67–8. You can use the same strategies at home: provide clean needles, food, clothing, and a bed. And, like Samantha, you can send your loved one to a harm reduction center to have their drugs tested and more. Here, we will focus on how you can inspire change.

Awakening the Motivation to Change

The opioid-addicted patients I see generally fall into one of three categories: the people who sit in my office by court order or some other force and want to keep using; those who recognize they have a problem and genuinely want help; and those who are apathetic—that is, they have lost interest in life, feel too defeated to care, or simply don't see their use as a big problem. All of them are scared stiff of going through withdrawal and keep using for now, as they cannot think of an alternative. Although not all of my patients are motivated to change when I first set eyes on them, most of them gradually desire to stop using and improve their life.

What happens between day one and the day a patient decides that not using is better than using? I do not wave some kind of magic wand. Along with many other therapists, I work toward one goal: to engage the person in thoughtful conversation in an effort to awaken their motivation to change.

Motivation isn't something you can pull out of a hat or command at will. It's internal, a drive that comes from within. Insisting that your loved one do things your way doesn't motivate. Addiction is too powerful against even the harshest words. Human nature at its core resists as well. In fact, these typical reactions do more harm than good: They push the person away. Consider the situation from the perspective of a person with OUD: After another blowup, your loved one—say, your son—decides not to come home. He is tired of hearing the lectures. Feeling judged, alone, and resentful, he does not speak up when he truly does want help. Who can he talk to? Who will understand? Anxious about all the strife in the house, he uses to ease his mind. He knows that what he is doing is hurting everyone he loves, including himself. He feels awful, a disgrace. And so he uses to feel better. It is the only way out.

Reprimands are the default, black-and-white response. Your loved one is wrong, you are right, and there is no in-between. So you hurl insults to get your point across. It's natural, this defense. It is also rooted in fear— you are scared to death about what is happening and how little control you have over it.

If "attacking" is the most intuitive but least helpful reaction, what would happen if you made a conscious effort to do the opposite? What if you supported your loved one so that they saw some hope? What if you had their trust, so that when they were ready, they came to you to seek help?

The approach is confusing for most people, who feel they are acting against their values. But look at it this way: I would wager that, deep down, nearly all opioid-addicted people reach a point where they want to end their misery and seek help. They just do not see how it is possible. Having someone in their corner supporting them, however, is like a ray of hope.

It may not seem fair, but the onus to create an environment for change falls on family and friends. Samantha was bound and determined to help Eric. She made a conscious decision to create a new normal. She cast aside the idea that her son was an ungrateful heroin user and accepted that he had a treatable disease and needed support. Instead of attacking Eric, Samantha opened up an honest and respectful conversation about opioid use with him—just as a therapist would. They talked. At first, their conversations were short and shallow. But Samantha's consistent, engaging approach left the doors open. More and more, Eric shared with his mom his feelings about using. She learned about how he hated what was happening to him, and she felt a shift. Eric was less secretive, more trusting. So was she.

What if you could do the same? It is not as if the opioid use is a secret. And if it is, it won't be for long. Imagine a calm, collected, mature conversation about what is going on in your addicted loved one's life. No judgment. Anger set aside. Just questions and answers. Empathy and compassion.

Lest this sound too unrealistic, let's compare this conversation to the "sex talk." Not talking about sex doesn't eliminate unsafe sex. Talking to your children about safe sex is the only way you learn how much they know about the subject. Your children may have sex whether you approve or not. If they trust you not to lose your mind if they tell you they are planning on or having a sexual relationship, you might have an opportunity to help them stay safe—or maybe get them to confess they are not ready. If you discover they are having sex, you can offer to buy condoms. You can also use the opportunity to set up some rules, such as that they need to see a doctor, practice effective birth control, do it in privacy, and cannot have sex when younger siblings are in the house. Avoiding the conversation about safe sex does not make sex safer for your children. Yelling and screaming closes the door to healthy conversation. The same holds true for drug use.

Your Strategy: Keep Asking the Right Questions

The idea is to ask insightful questions—about your loved one's life, use, concerns—so they see for themselves that what they are doing conflicts with their true goals. You repeatedly engage your loved one in respectful, empathetic conversation, and in doing so earn their trust. These conversations lead to self-awareness and, ultimately, the desire to change.

Motivational interviewing is fairly simple under normal circumstances. But addiction in the household doesn't feel anything close to normal, and, under duress, it is tempting to criticize and blame. Avoid these kinds of jabs. Postpone your talk if you are feeling vulnerable or angry. Your questions and remarks should show your loved one that you empathize with them. You want to understand where they are coming from.

Once you understand the framework and the steps needed to ask the right questions in the right way, you will see how everything falls into place. Yet, because motivational interviewing is based on conversation, it is a dynamic process. It goes back and forth. One day you will think you have made great progress, and the next day you are back where you started. What prevails throughout, however, is that you talk to your loved one. When you keep the conversation open, the person with addiction feels less ambivalent about seeking help. You focus on their strengths and respect their autonomy. Over time, you earn their trust as someone who will not judge them.

An Added Benefit

Motivational interviewing comes with some additional perks: it also helps you.

When you are hopeless, when you don't know what to do, when you are stuck, you likely get angry. Anger is a huge element when dealing with an addicted family member. When angry, people tend to do one of two things: withdraw in defiance or lash out. Neither response is usually helpful. Not talking creates more distance. When lashing out, the tendency is to demean the person: call them names, label them, or tell them how worthless they are. This helps you release your anger but settles nothing. You are left to regurgitate your negative thoughts, over and over for hours on end, which only brings you further down. And feeling your wrath does little to help the addicted individual change. They are already very hard on themselves. They already know and believe what you are

Tips

If you feel too angry or emotional, walk away. Save the conversation for another time. You are not angry all the time. You have moments when you feel tender and more accepting, so wait for those moments. Think about couples. When they are angry, they don't talk about complicated problems. They have to take care of themselves. If you don't know what to do, take care of yourself. Physically and mentally. Get your needs met. Connect with people who can give you strength.

Do it in small steps. Making a small change is better than no change. Ask: Can we agree on something? Can you be positive about some small change? Can you commit to not hanging out with such and such? Can you be respectful? Come up with something small that is acceptable to both sides. In making small changes, you feel a sense of accomplishment, which serves as encouragement to continue.

Be consistent and persistent. Keep buying the needles, even when you feel you have not made progress. At times, you might feel beat up in the process, but you must be persistent. Switching your strategy to one of punishment, for instance, will only cause you to lose a lot of the trust you have worked hard to earn. Likewise, be consistently firm with your family rules.

Get help for yourself. Addiction's toll on a family gets worse before it gets better. Even when a loved one is in recovery, family members need help. Don't underestimate how important self-care is for you and other family members. Reach out to others for support. Find a counselor, attend a family program for addiction (some treatment centers open their family progams up to the general public), or attend Al-Anon or Nar-Anon groups. If you are unable to deal with an addicted family member, see whether you can get your loved one to see a therapist, who can keep the conversation open.

telling them. When you face the truth calmly and with compassion, you rise above your negative thoughts, worry, and anxiety. You feel you are making progress, making a positive difference. For the first time in a long time, you feel good.

If your loved one is addicted to opioids, eventually they will experience some of the negative consequences of using. When they do, you will want to have kept the conversation open so that they will turn to you and be able to ask for help. When they do, you will be ready.

Your Role as Interviewer

Let's take a closer look at why something so simple as asking questions can motivate someone to change. Motivational interviewing is a strategy developed by Drs. William R. Miller and Stephen Rollnick that helps people recognize and do something about their problem. It is a unique style of talking to individuals who use substances. It has three main characteristics:

- Collaboration versus confrontation—you work with rather than against.
- Evocation versus education—you encourage conversation rather than teach.
- Autonomy versus authoritarianism—you respect independence rather than try to control.

Collaboration

Motivational interviewing is rooted in the spirit of *collaboration*—not confrontation. You talk to your loved one about their substance use. You voice an openness to change by asking open-ended questions: *What do opioids do for you? How do you feel when you can't take them? What happens during withdrawal? I know it's difficult; it looks like you're struggling. I want to know how to help. Tell me what I can do for you.*

When you take on a peer-like role of adviser, you give your loved one permission to tell you things they might otherwise hold back. You elicit

Conversation Starters

You can open up an honest conversation by asking questions about what you can do to help. Avoid digging for details and inciting confrontation. The questions you ask—and the answers you get—will depend in part on the relationship you have with your addicted loved one. They might respond defensively or be guarded. They might break down and cry. Or they might start talking and ask for help. Regardless, show them that you are there to help in any way possible, to understand, and to empathize—not to judge. And avoid confrontation completely. Walk away when you start feeling like you are no longer working toward the same goal. If these questions feel contrived, change them to sound more natural for you, but keep the objective in mind: You are trying to engage your loved one by showing your support.

- What do opioids do for you? How do they make you feel?
- What do you use, how much, and how often? Where do you get it?
- How do you feel when you don't take them?
- Do you always feel good when you get high?
- Are there any tough moments?
- Are there things you wish you did not have to go through?
- Do you inject? Do you sometimes use dirty needles?
- I see that you're struggling. How can I help you?

their point of view. You are truly interested in what they want out of life, in knowing what they value, and how they want their life to look. You are not concerned with educating them about how bad they've been. Your main concern is to keep the conversation open and work together toward the same goal, which is to make things better.

Evocation

Feeling heard and understood is sometimes the most powerful medicine. The addicted person lets down their guard and starts thinking about the possibilities. You help them *evoke* memories and images of how they want their life to look and feel. They see the large discrepancies between how they want to live and how they are living. As they do this, feelings of motivation begin to stir within, even if ever so slightly.

Autonomy

All the while, you allow the addicted person to live their life as they must. You give them *autonomy*—they control their actions and you support their choices—to a point. This does not mean they can do whatever they want to you and your family. They do not get to wrap you around their finger. You are supportive and nonjudgmental, consistent, trustworthy, reliable, calm, and cool, but you stand behind established limits—that is, you have your boundaries. For example: *You can live here but don't ask me for money for drugs. If you try to intimidate me, you need to leave. You cannot curse me out. I expect you to be respectful. Threatening behavior of any kind, to anyone in this house, is unacceptable.* Be as specific as possible: *Curfew is 11:00 p.m. If you come home later, the rest of us lie awake fearing the worst.*

The person who uses drugs has the right to use—which is something they feel they cannot deny themselves—provided they heed their known limits about using in the house or leaving tainted needles lying around. Because both of you know that they use, you are free to offer clean needles, a roof over their head, or a hot meal. You do not dictate how the addicted individual lives, but you protect yourself and your family as best you can by setting and standing by limits. This approach leaves little room for resentment—how can this person resent you for letting them live their life?

These conversations are not intuitive. Speaking in this way requires you to give up the idea of being right and foster as much empathy as possible—even as the addicted loved one tears your heart out. It requires trusting someone who has repeatedly betrayed your trust in the past. But it is effective. The worst thing you can do is not talk to your loved one, which only further alienates them. Now they are not only using but angry. Genuine conversation leads to impact, and you must bend over backward to keep the conversation open. If you are not in the habit of speaking to your loved one this way when you are hurt and angry, you will be pleasantly surprised when you see how they respond and how much better you feel.

Motivation Versus the Traditional "Rock Bottom"

"Hitting bottom" is the traditional way to enter treatment: The consequences of using are so bad that the addicted person is finally motivated enough to surrender. While this can work with some addictions, it is risky with opioid addiction. With the strength of the opioids available today, all too often rock bottom is the final consequence.

Capture your audience while you can. Talk, listen, understand, and make every effort to earn your loved one's trust. When they are ready to

Signs and Symptoms of Opioid Intoxication

Most people who use opioids look normal. Or they might look a little loopy or animated or be in too good a mood. People who are physically dependent on opioids try to take enough drugs to keep themselves comfortable, but if they take too much, they get sleepy, or "nod off." If they don't have enough, they are irritable. Other signs and symptoms include:

- Slurred speech
- Decreased responsiveness
- Apathy
- Slow and shallow breathing
- Cold, clammy skin
- Small or pinpoint pupils

make a change—and at some point they will be ready—you'll be there to take their hand and help them to do what they cannot do for themselves.

Samantha had a lofty goal. It was not to keep Eric using. Her goal was to get him to stop. And she planned to do it first by doing all she could to keep Eric alive and second by establishing herself as an advocate rather than an enemy. Talking to him, asking him what he was going through and what opioids did for him, lending an ear, and listening to his struggles—empathizing. To Eric, his mom became someone he knew he could turn to for help. Someone he could talk to without feeling judged, without fear of punishment. Someone who would be there for him if he overdosed, ready to give him lifesaving medicine. Samantha had earned Eric's trust. And when he hit another low—severe withdrawal—and was feeling most vulnerable, he was ready to start talking about treatment.

House Rules

We respect your need to use. In turn, we expect you to respect our decisions about what we will allow in our household. The following is not allowed:

- Using drugs in the house
- Threatening or intimidating anyone for money or drugs
- Stealing
- Coming home after 11:00 p.m.
- Leaving used needles around the house
- Leaving drugs or medication where your siblings can access them

If any of these rules is broken, we need to discuss whether you can continue to live at home.

A Mother's Story

While Michael (whose story begins in chapter 3) is in treatment, his parents attend the center's family program. JoAnn, his mom, describes how the four-day program changed her view of addiction forever. "I learned a lot. The neurologist explained how the brain works and how people react differently to drugs. I found it fascinating. This resonated with me. I will never again look at addiction as something people really choose to do."

JoAnn also notices a common theme: Everyone in the program confesses that they kept their loved one's addiction a secret for as long as possible. During the worst of times, no one shared their struggles. "I did the same thing until I started getting sick to my stomach. I realized I can't keep this in. I started talking to friends. If anyone had a problem with it, I cut them off. I didn't need judgment. Addiction can happen to anyone. I saw this at the center—people from good backgrounds, older people, businesspeople, moms."

Signs and Symptoms of Withdrawal

People addicted to opioids spend the majority of their addicted lives not enjoying a high but attempting to feel "normal" or avoiding withdrawal—what they call being "dope sick." Compared to withdrawal from other drugs, opioid withdrawal can be extremely uncomfortable but not usually life threatening. The severity of withdrawal symptoms depends on many factors, including whether the person took high doses, more frequent doses, or injected; the length of time that has passed since the last dose; and whether other drugs were taken. It is also greater if the person takes short-acting opioids, such as heroin. Withdrawal can be mild and almost unnoticeable or quite severe and obvious to everyone around. Some people can look very sick but not complain much, whereas others have no clear signs of withdrawal but complain a lot. The only way to avoid the symptoms of withdrawal is to take more opioids. Users can reduce some symptoms by taking over-the-counter medications.

The most common withdrawal symptoms include:

- Anxiety
- Irritability
- Feeling restless, especially in legs
- Cold sweats and shaking chills
- Watery eyes/runny nose
- Large pupils
- Yawning
- Muscle aches in back and legs
- Stomach cramps
- No appetite

More severe withdrawal includes:

- Nausea and vomiting
- Diarrhea
- Leg and arm muscle spasms ("kicking the habit")
- Gooseflesh on forearms ("cold turkey")
- Fever
- Severe insomnia
- Confusion and disorientation

After the acute withdrawal resolves, usually within five to seven days, some people may continue to experience withdrawal-like symptoms that can last for many weeks. This set of symptoms is called "protracted withdrawal" and may include:

- Anxiety
- Irritability
- Feelings of sadness
- Inability to enjoy anything
- Mood swings
- Feeling stressed
- Poor sleep
- Cravings for opioids

JoAnn's saving grace has been her support system—her husband and two other sons, a long list of nonjudgmental friends, and God. "My faith really kicked in. I kept praying. I still pray a lot. Anyone who goes through this must, must, must have a great support system at home. I wouldn't have made it without it."

How to Help an Opioid User Through Withdrawal

Withdrawal is perhaps the most feared word in an opioid user's vocabulary. Fear of going through withdrawal likely keeps more people out of treatment than finances or long waiting lists, which is why educating opioid users about methadone and buprenorphine is so important. Withdrawal is what happens to the bodies of daily opioid users when their drug of choice is either not consumed or taken in smaller quantities than usual. Going through withdrawal is another way of talking about detoxing off opioids.

Your loved one may have on more than one occasion decided to stop using opioids and go "cold turkey," or detox at home with no medications. I would estimate that 99 percent of the time, opioid withdrawal is not dangerous, unlike like alcohol withdrawal, which in severe cases can lead to confusion, high body temperature, seizures, and death (delirium tremens, aka the DTs). Opioid withdrawal is highly uncomfortable but self-limiting. It usually comes on gradually, is most severe one to two days after the last dose, and resolves gradually in five to seven days. Withdrawal symptoms will stop on their own.

Withdrawal is best done under a doctor's supervision using prescription medications, but most people actually go through opioid withdrawal on their own at home. Most people can do this safely, provided they follow a few simple rules. Ideally, they will have a family member with them or a medical professional checking on them frequently. Going through withdrawal in the hospital is always a good idea, but this option may not be available to everyone because of cost or accessibility. If your loved one becomes confused, disoriented, or unable to respond during withdrawal (which is rare), falls and hits their head, or has a medical illness and goes into withdrawal, take them immediately to the ER, where they can get more advanced medical attention.

Otherwise, do your best to respect your loved one's wishes, short of supplying them with opioids. Withdrawal is a negative consequence of opioid addiction. While you don't want them to suffer, *you are not responsible for supplying them with drugs.* If they want a medically supervised withdrawal in the hospital, which is far more comfortable than white-knuckling it, take them to the ER. If they prefer to detox at home, help keep them as comfortable as possible. Treat them as you would treat someone who has a severe flu. Being well hydrated is the key to making withdrawal more tolerable. Keep a glass of water at bedside at all times. Stock plenty of sports drinks or fluid replacement drinks made for children (such as Pedialyte) to replace electrolytes, as well as broth or chocolate milk for easily digestible nourishment. Avoid serving your loved one regular food for a few days. Stick with crackers and other easily digestible snacks.

Medications used during withdrawal to counteract specific symptoms may not shorten withdrawal but will make it much less severe, encouraging the person to stick with the plan to detoxify rather than go back to using opioids. It is rare for someone to die from opioid withdrawal itself (although people might feel as if they are going to die), but if your loved one has a chronic or preexisting illness, such as high blood pressure, asthma, or diabetes, you will want to take precautions. Likewise, if they have an active infection, flu, pneumonia, or acute hepatitis, or a serious injury, going through withdrawal should be postponed or done under medical supervision. In withdrawal, the body goes through a state of intense arousal and major stress. Already-weak organs may fail when stressed. In the case of diabetes, for instance, the pancreas may shut down, causing sugar levels to shoot up and put the person who is withdrawing in a diabetic coma.

Over-the-counter medications can relieve most of the symptoms. Have handy products that relieve diarrhea, nausea, and vomiting; antacids to counteract stomach pain; as well as remedies for muscle pain, sleep, and anxiety.

The Only Reason to Go Through Withdrawal

People put themselves through opioid withdrawal either because they do not have any opioids or intentionally as a first step toward quitting opioids altogether. *The only reason your loved one should go through withdrawal is if they are planning to start relapse prevention treatment with naltrexone.* Detoxification is very dangerous otherwise. Going through withdrawal, or detoxing off opioids, is not by itself a treatment for OUD. Completing withdrawal will not "cure" OUD. A great majority of people who finish detoxing will relapse and use opioids again. However, OUD treatment medication decreases the risk of relapse. If your loved one goes through withdrawal because they cannot get drugs, it is an opportunity to talk to them about treatment. Once they've detoxed, they can start naltrexone. Or, if they do not want to face a week or more of withdrawal symptoms, they can start methadone or buprenorphine.

People who detox and do not continue treatment with medications are vulnerable to overdose. Only a small percentage die, but there is no way to tell who will fall within that statistic. Medication reduces the risk of overdose many times over. Withdrawal is an opportunity to talk about treatment options and take action. Every crisis is an opportunity for change, because people in crisis are often willing to accept help. Suffering through withdrawal is often a wake-up call. So is overdosing.

Dealing with Overdose

Overdose is common in people who use opioids. Some are more likely to overdose than others. Most often, overdose happens when a person starts using again after a period of abstinence—after returning home from an inpatient detox unit or a residential treatment program that does not use medication to treat OUD. It happens to people released from prison or college students returning home for a break. We do not know why some overdose repeatedly and others never do. We know that people with a history of overdose are six times more likely to overdose again. Injecting opioids and combining them with alcohol or sedative drugs, such as Xanax, also increases that risk.

911 Good Samaritan and Naloxone Access Laws

All fifty states have Good Samaritan laws that protect people who try to help victims of a car accident or administer CPR in a medical emergency, for example. If something goes wrong, the helpful citizen is generally protected from legal consequences. The idea is to encourage bystanders to help in emergencies. While all states have Good Samaritan laws, not all of them are created equal.

As of this writing, forty states as well as the District of Columbia have additional provisions to protect those who report or experience drug overdoses or who administer naloxone to the overdose victim. The drug overdose immunity laws are a legislative effort to encourage people to seek help for an overdose victim. Although the laws vary, many states even protect the caller or the overdose victim from being arrested for outstanding legal issues. However, if the victim or the caller is on probation or parole, these protections may not be offered. The idea is to prevent death from overdose and, in some states, shepherd the person who has overdosed into treatment—not the legal system. Check the Good Samaritan laws in your state. Hopefully, all states will soon offer full legal protections to all lay people who want to use naloxone to save lives.

Most overdoses are not lethal. Emergency medical staff manages half of them, while the other half are self-managed by family or friends. Fewer than 5 percent of them end in death. In most people, overdose is not instant. Death comes after minutes or even hours of gradually slowing respirations. More often than not, there is time to reverse the overdose before it can result in death. Sometimes, when help comes a bit late, the lack of oxygen to the brain results in permanent neurological damage. But often, breathing can be restored in time for a complete recovery with no lasting damage.

Signs and Symptoms of an Opioid Overdose

There is a fine line between being really high and overdosing. If someone is really high (but not overdosing), they will respond to outside stimuli, such as a loud noise or touch. If overdosing, they will have a pulse and take occasional breaths but will not respond or wake up to a painful stimulation.

Other overdose symptoms include:

- Slow, shallow, or irregular breathing
- Lips and fingernails turn bluish-purple or gray
- Skin is pale and clammy to the touch
- Pupils are pinpoint and react to light; in severe cases, pupils are large and do not react to light
- Choking sounds (death rattle)
- Frothing at the mouth

Not everyone is comfortable responding to a life-threatening overdose. Always call 911. And do your best to create a network of support people who are comfortable helping—neighbors, friends, and relatives. Families cannot afford to keep opioid addiction a secret. When your goal is to do everything in your power to keep your loved one alive, secrets can be deadly.

Naloxone (Narcan): The New Normal

Many a heroin user has been force-fed, had ice-cold water thrown on their genitals, been slapped hard across a cheek, or even injected with milk to bring them out of an opioid overdose. This was common in the past, but things have changed. A cheap and highly effective antidote to overdose called naloxone, better known by its brand name, Narcan, is now widely available, so much so that stocking it in the kitchen cupboard has become the new normal.

Friends, relatives, or even strangers may witness an overdose. Witnesses who have access to naloxone and know how to use it can save lives. Overdose-reversal kits can be purchased at the local pharmacy in communities where a health-care commissioner has issued a community-wide prescription. Where this is not available, a family doctor can prescribe naloxone. In either case, the pharmacist will dispense the naloxone, no questions asked. The pharmacist will not usually provide training on how to use it, although some preparations of naloxone may include instructions in their packaging materials. Another way to get kits is to attend overdose-prevention trainings for families. These trainings exist in a few states, run by either the Department of Health or a grassroots organization. If your loved one is in treatment, the program should offer trainings and dispense naloxone to family members. If they don't, ask for it. Patients receiving painkillers should be given naloxone as an antidote. Again, ask for it.

Naloxone is safe and easy to use, and most of the time administering it to a person suffering an opioid overdose can reverse the overdose before permanent damage occurs. Learning how to perform CPR may prove to be an added benefit, as opioids can stop an overdose victim from breathing. So, I will go so far as to say that everyone who lives with or is in regular contact with a person who uses opioids, or has painkillers in the house—*whether addiction is present or not*—should be sure they:

- Know how to recognize an overdose
- Stock at least one overdose-reversal kit in the home and/or car

- Are comfortable using the kit to reverse an overdose
- Are prepared to call 911

Like it or not, this is the new normal. The good thing is that administering naloxone is not as hard as you might think. Here are the steps you need to be aware of:

1. Confirm that the person has overdosed on opioids: They do not wake up, are not breathing, or are breathing really slowly (about one breath every five or more seconds); have blue or gray lips and fingernails and pale or clammy skin.
2. Use your knuckles to rub the person's sternum (the hard bone in the middle of the chest), to try to rouse them.
3. If they do not wake up, call 911 and say you may have an opioid overdose victim.
4. Give naloxone according to your training or the instructions on the package. You may have a naloxone injection or a nasal spray. If you have a spray, simply remove the spray from its package, insert it fully in the victim's nose with their head tilted back, and press the plunger firmly until all medication is released. If you have an injection kit, open the cap on the naloxone vial, insert the provided syringe with needle into the vial, draw all the naloxone from the vial (1 cc), pull it out, expose the person's skin on their upper arm, thigh, or buttock, quickly insert the needle deep into the muscle in the selected area, and push the whole content of the syringe into the muscle over a few seconds. The order of Steps 3 and 4 can be reversed. If someone else is with you, one of you can call 911 while the other administers naloxone.
5. It may take one to three minutes for the naloxone to start working. If the person's chest does not rise and fall with respirations, perform mouth-to-mouth resuscitation to prevent brain damage while you wait for the naloxone to start working.

6. If you see no effect in three to five minutes and the individual is still unconscious and not breathing, take out another dose of naloxone and repeat. You want to see breathing restored. The person does not need to be fully alert. If their chest does not rise and fall with respirations, continue to perform mouth-to-mouth resuscitation while you wait for the ambulance.

7. After you give naloxone and the person starts breathing, keep them calm, do not let them use again, and stay with them until the paramedics arrive. If you cannot wait because you are afraid of getting arrested, leave the person in a stable position on their side. Bend their top knee and ensure both arms are positioned in the same direction as the top knee. Leave the space around their nose and mouth clear so they do not choke if they vomit. Leave the naloxone packaging nearby so paramedics will see what medication has been administered.

8. Naloxone wears off in thirty to ninety minutes, and breathing may stop again. Overdose victims need to go to the emergency room for further treatment and observation. It is possible to deliver too little naloxone, so call 911 if you have not yet done so.

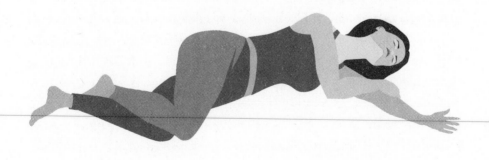

Dos and Don'ts of Opioid Overdose Reversal

Do always call 911 or take the overdose victim to the ER after administering naloxone. Paramedics may give the person oxygen to assist their breathing. Hospital staff will monitor the patient for at least a few hours, measure oxygen levels, and readminister naloxone as necessary. Professionals will evaluate the individual for addiction and may even offer treatment on the spot. Your loved one may be receptive to treatment in this time of crisis.

Do administer naloxone even though the person might have overdosed on other drugs. Sometimes fentanyl can be present in fake sedatives (e.g., fake Xanax bars) or even cocaine. Naloxone will not reverse overdose on sedatives, sleeping pills, cocaine, or alcohol, but if the person overdosed on a combination of drugs, it may be enough to bring their breathing back.

Do administer additional doses of naloxone if the first one does not produce any effects. The person might have overdosed on a fentanyl-like substance, which is a very powerful opioid. Naloxone in usual doses may not be sufficient to counteract fentanyl, methadone, or injected buprenorphine, so it is important that you give more than one dose if you have it. There is little harm from giving too much naloxone if the person is not breathing, but not giving enough can lead to death or permanent brain damage.

Do get certified to provide mouth-to-mouth resuscitation/CPR to supplement breathing. If the person is not breathing and you are waiting for naloxone to start working or you have no more naloxone to give, you can do mouth-to-mouth resuscitation to give the overdose victim some oxygen. Basically, you lay the person flat on their back, tilt their head back, check that there is nothing in their mouth, and pinch their nose shut. Using a mouth barrier (which can be purchased at any drugstore and prevents the spread of HIV) or not, cover their mouth with your lips and blow air in, as many times as you can, giving one breath every five seconds. Short training sessions on resuscitation are available in most clinical settings for a nominal fee, and many employers offer courses for free.

Don't administer naloxone unless the person has overdosed. If they are only sleepy from having too much heroin and you give them naloxone, you will cancel their high and put them in the very unpleasant state of withdrawal. When in doubt, however, do administer the naloxone, as withdrawal is better than brain damage.

Don't give naloxone to someone who is awake and breathing normally. This can put them in severe withdrawal and injure the lungs.

When you suspect a child has been exposed to opioids

Opioid overdose can happen to anyone who takes opioids, including children who accidently swallow a painkiller or touch heroin powder. More than one parent has come across a child who is not responding because of an accidental overdose. You should call 911, but it may take too long for first responders to arrive. Overdose reversal needs to happen as soon as possible, within minutes for powerful opioids such as fentanyl. Overdose reversal kits work the same for children as they do for adults, though the dose may be too high for children. If you suspect overdose in a child, it is best to first call 911, describe the situation, tell them that you have naloxone, and wait for their instructions. You may also administer mouth-to-mouth resuscitation to a child, but your breaths will be lighter than they are for adults. Infants, especially, can only handle so much air in their lungs. I recommend resuscitation training for all parents who have opioids and children in the house.

When Talking Isn't Enough

Motivational interviewing is one of several effective approaches to inspire your loved one to get help. I also recommend a more formalized method of working with a drug-using family member called community reinforcement and family training (CRAFT), which involves the entire family as well as friends. CRAFT teaches people how to interact with the addicted individual. As with motivational interviewing, the idea is to reduce harm and keep inching the loved one with a drug problem toward treatment. A big piece of CRAFT is improving the lives of everyone involved with the person struggling with addiction, especially family members. CRAFT is not specific to opioid addiction, but the methods apply. And CRAFT success rates are quite high.

Staging an intervention is another option, especially when there is an urgent concern about your loved one's safety and other methods of getting help have not worked. You can hire a professional interventionist who instructs family and friends to write honest letters to the addicted individual and conducts a meeting. Each person at the intervention lovingly reads their letter to the addicted person (who is caught off guard). A daughter, for instance, might describe how empty she feels when her dad doesn't show up for her baseball games or her embarrassment when Dad stumbles in front of her friends.

Interventions can and do work for many people, but if they backfire, the person who is sitting center stage feels completely alienated. Instead of taking a step forward, you have taken many steps back. When interventions work, an added benefit is that everything is planned—from a reserved room at a select treatment center to the airplane tickets and packed bags, leaving little time or opportunity for the individual to change their mind. Interventions can work at times of crisis, when the addicted person may be desperate for a solution and ready to accept it. But before you schedule an intervention, I recommend that you first meet with an addiction psychologist or physician to discuss whether other options might be available. You might want to try a CRAFT strategy first before organizing an intervention.

When to Call in the Troops

I have given you a tall order in this chapter. What I'm asking you to do is not for the faint of heart. On paper, it might sound straightforward. But real life has a way of showing us that things aren't always as simple as they sound. Addiction is called a family disease because it affects everyone in the household. The person with addiction gets all the attention (albeit negative). Parents have much less time to tend to other children or their spouses. Feeling ignored, children act out. Parents or spouses spend an inordinate amount of time worrying and isolating. Too ashamed to talk about the family problem or too stressed to want to talk, adults abandon relationships with friends and family. Work suffers, as one family member or another must tend to another crisis—bailing their son out of jail or picking up a husband from the ER postoverdose. Everyone walks on eggshells. And it never ends. The worry, fear, crises. It never ends and as the addiction gets stronger, the family gets weaker, less sure of itself, and easily thrown into a rapidly descending whirlpool of lies and confusion.

When you feel you are not the one to help your loved one, you can help yourself. If you are too lost in the person's behavior, you can't control your anger, you can't think straight, or the addiction has gone on for too long and taken too large a toll on you, work with a therapist. In therapy, you can acknowledge all the feelings of anger, hopelessness, powerlessness, failure, fear—all of these legitimate feelings that surface when you are dealing with an impossible situation. Even one session with a therapist can sometimes put years of emotional pain into perspective and even offer ways to bring out feelings of compassion and acceptance to replace harmful negative emotions.

The Beauty Behind Preparation

Samantha was prepared. She had read as much about opioids, addiction, and overdose as she could. She attended an overdose reversal training and took a resuscitation class. She kept a steady supply of clean needles and condoms for her son, as well as over-the-counter medications to help with withdrawal. She walked tall when confronted with backlash from family and turned to her supports when it became too overwhelming. On the side of her refrigerator hung a list of emergency phone numbers, including nearby detox centers, hospitals, harm reduction centers, personal contacts, and select treatment centers. She updated it as needed. Samantha also met with a local addiction professional, so she knew about all treatment options and which places offered the kind of treatment Eric needed. When Eric could not find the money he needed to buy drugs and started going through withdrawal, she was at his side, helping him through his misery. Twenty-four hours later, Eric confided that he was ready to seek help.

Samantha was ready, too.

CHAPTER 9

Finding the Right Treatment

When George first seeks treatment for opioid addiction, he is taking ten to fifteen oxycodone pills a day, all of which he buys on the black market. His use began five years earlier, after he was injured on the job when some materials fell from a building at a construction site and landed on his right foot. Three broken toes and some crushed tissue left him with significant bruising, swelling, and pain. The doctor could do only so much. Healing would take place on its own, in time. The doctor taped George's toes, gave him a two-week prescription for oxycodone, and sent him on his merry way. When George needed more painkillers, the doctor wrote another prescription. This went on for about three years—long after George had healed and no longer felt pain from the injury. George knew he was taking the pills for other reasons, namely to cope with a stressful job and an increasingly difficult marriage, but he didn't want to admit it. At the three-year mark, however, the doctor started weaning George off opioids, at first giving him pills of lower dosages and then fewer pills.

George seemed to be doing well, but that was because, through his co-workers, he had found another source of painkillers. For about one year, he bought his pills through co-workers and eventually the black market, spending about $30 a pop—eventually about $400 a day. George made good money, but he also had a wife and three children to support. He hated diverting all the money away from his family, but he was so preoccupied with getting more pills and avoiding withdrawal that he couldn't seem to stop. If he did stop, he felt anxious and couldn't sleep. Before long, his guilt over spending all that money on illegal drugs weighed heavily on his conscience. He just couldn't do it anymore.

A lot of the guys he worked with used opioids, but that also meant that some were in treatment. George discreetly asked around and heard about Suboxone. The drug, a combination of buprenorphine and naloxone, contains a small bit of an opioid, but it works differently than oxycodone. People do not need higher and higher doses, and it reduces cravings and prevents overdose. One guy told George that it worked great for him—he didn't have cravings and was no longer spending all his time and money on drugs. "Google 'Suboxone treatment,'" said the colleague. "You can find someone who can prescribe it in your town."

George went to the psychiatrist he found online, told his story, and said that he wanted to try Suboxone. After completing an evaluation, the doctor diagnosed George with moderate opioid use disorder (OUD) and explained George's treatment options. She also thought Suboxone would work for George, who was motivated and ready to make a change.

"It was easy," George remembers. "I went through a little withdrawal before the first dose, but once I started taking it, I quickly felt better. No withdrawal symptoms, no drug cravings, nothing. It was like I didn't skip a beat, yet everything got so much better."

The psychiatrist initially placed George on a high dose—three strips a day—and gradually decreased it over the course of a few years to a half strip per day. George did great. His symptoms went away and his life improved. Then he had another accident and was offered pain medication in the hospital. Hearing the offer, and being in severe pain, his addictive thinking took over.

"I should have told them I was on Suboxone, but I didn't. There was a part of me that didn't really want to admit I was an addict. I guess in some way I was embarrassed, ashamed that I was an addict. Thought I wouldn't be treated the same way. Another part of me was thinking, here I have a chance to get pills for free. And it is legitimate. So, I went home with a bottle of painkillers."

George stopped taking Suboxone and took the painkillers instead. "I knew better, but I did it because they were there." As if not wanting to be wasteful, he went through all the pills. When the prescription ran out, George was scared. He didn't want to fall back into the same useless, unending cycle. He called his psychiatrist and told her he had relapsed. "She wasn't upset or judgmental. She said it was part of the process and asked me to come back. This was a huge relief. I was feeling guilty enough as it was."

After his brief relapse, George remembers what he is like when he is using. "I had a lot more conflict in my life when I was on pills. I was irritable and quickly got upset, especially with my wife. We'd argue a lot, and we did not have sex for months. And I had no patience for my children. I still had my job—otherwise I wouldn't have been able to buy the drugs. I mostly hurt my family by not being there and wasting so much money. And I hated lying to them. I had to hide a lot and that did not feel good."

George can't imagine what life would be like if he hadn't gotten on Suboxone. "Till this day, I wonder what would have happened if I'd lost the house or my wife or been arrested or overdosed. I don't even want to go there. I have friends who I see are struggling, and it makes me wonder if I would still have my family. But my marriage is better than ever. I open up with the doc and talk about difficult decisions. That helps me deal with stress."

If George doesn't take his medication on time, he starts feeling antsy. That is his only side effect, yet it is also a gentle reminder. He used to see his psychiatrist once a month, then every two months. Now, he goes four to five times a year, mostly to talk about what might be stressing him out. He knows that uncomfortable and unaddressed feelings, or getting on a wrong train of thought, can lead him back to pills. He never goes to any other type of therapy. Although he checked out a local AA meeting once, he decided it was not useful for him and never went back.

George's worries now center on what would happen if he were seriously injured again and needed painkillers.

"I do worry about having a big car accident or something. What would I do for the pain? Now, I would tell the ER docs. I would tell them about my addiction. I hope they would know what to do."

Barriers to Seeking Treatment

What happened with George is not only a true but a very common scenario. I would estimate that the type of low-level care he received would make a huge difference for about one quarter of the 2.4 million people suffering from OUD. Fear and confusion, however, get in the way.

The Georges of the world are the easiest to treat. Most primary care doctors, nurse practitioners, and physician assistants would be able to handle his case quite easily, without further referrals. Recovery required little effort on George's part. George wasn't doing crazy stuff. He smoked cigarettes and drank but was not injecting heroin or using other illegal drugs. He held a job and kept his marriage together. He was able to hide his addiction from his wife, who thought he was just overstressed. Yet he clearly has OUD.

A lot of people like George are maintained on painkillers for years and not doing well. They are injured on the job, get workers' compensation insurance, and stay at home. They take their painkillers, drink beer, watch television, and get depressed. They could feel much better if they were diagnosed with OUD and on proper treatment, but they do not know their options. They are afraid, really terrified, of giving up pills, and this prevents them from seeking help.

Another barrier is confusion about pathways into treatment. People will tell you they have tried to get into treatment, but it was too complicated. They did not know where to start, what to expect, or whether they could afford it. Even methadone clinics proved problematic. They had to apply and wait days, even weeks, before knowing whether they were accepted—and that is more than long enough to find a reason to postpone treatment again. If they called a treatment center, their name was added to a long wait list or they were asked to call back in a day or two. But many people with addiction don't have a change of clothing, much less a phone. And they certainly don't have time. If they think about it for too long, the next call they make will be to their dealer.

As of this writing, finding help is more complicated than it should be, but if you start by considering what is most important, the path suddenly becomes clear. People like George benefit from understanding how simple treatment can be. The day George's foot was injured affected his life, and it could have destroyed it if he had not gotten help. More severe cases of OUD might require swifter action—perhaps getting the addicted person on overdose prevention medication before he changes his mind about treatment or he needs to use again.

In this chapter, I have outlined various avenues that you can take to help your loved one or yourself, but almost all roads to recovery from opioids can start with buprenorphine. So your first question shouldn't be *Where do I go for help?* but *Who offers buprenorphine?*

Let's look at why buprenorphine can be so crucial.

Buprenorphine: Medication That Buys You Time

When people who use opioids are ready for treatment, there is little time to waste. Another hour or two, and they have changed their minds. It is not that they are fickle. Their brains are calling for more opioids, and at those moments, logic takes a backseat. Knowing your options ahead of time—before your loved one is ready—can save you some grief.

When Eric (the story from chapter 7) asked for help, Samantha put her plan in motion. She called the family doctor and got Eric into their clinic the same day. Dr. Harrison, who was already familiar with the family struggles from having spoken with Samantha, talked to Eric briefly about his use and his health, quickly examined him, took his vitals, did a urine drug test in the office, and wrote a prescription for buprenorphine. She gave Eric instructions about when to take his first dose at home, prepared him for what to expect, and suggested he follow up with her on the phone the next day and again in two or three days. Eric scheduled an appointment to come into the office in a week to see how it was going. At that point, they would decide next steps.

If you recall from chapter 4, buprenorphine is a partial opioid agonist. It blocks some of the opioid receptor sites in the brain, preventing the patient from getting too high and overdosing. It also circumvents withdrawal and alleviates opioid cravings. The patient does not need to be completely detoxed before starting buprenorphine, which means it can be taken by people who are actively using, ready for help, and will do anything to avoid going through withdrawal. After an overnight abstinence, the patient is in mild withdrawal, the signal to take the first dose. In a few hours the patient starts feeling normal. By the end of that same day, most of these patients feel surprisingly well given that they have not taken their usual dose of heroin or painkillers.

For a select group of patients with OUD, a brief evaluation with a physician and a prescription for buprenorphine is all it takes. *That is all it takes.* They only need to take buprenorphine for a few days before they find they can think and function again. For many, many other people, the medicine buys time—enough so they can undergo a thorough assessment and decide next steps, which may or may not include buprenorphine.

In addition to possibly preventing an overdose or other disaster, buprenorphine is equally important because it puts your loved one in the treatment system. Once in the system, they will be directed to all the services and supports they need. Neither of you has to go around dazed and confused, trying to figure out where to get help. Your only job from this point onward in terms of finding services is to ensure you approve of the treatment services being offered. (On page 188 in this chapter, you'll find a program scorecard you can use to evaluate services.)

This scenario may be seen as too good to be true, and in some cases it is. Most medical professionals are not treating patients addicted to opioids. They may not be certified, may feel they do not have enough training, or may be reluctant to take on this new group of potentially difficult patients. Some doctors have had a bad experience treating people for opioid addiction and now feel prejudiced. Some OUD patients are complicated—they may present with other psychiatric disorders, use other drugs, or have many social problems that need to be addressed. Also, patients can get in their own way—they may be reluctant to start taking medications because they heard they are addictive or that they will need to take them for the rest of their lives. These barriers prevent many people from getting started with buprenorphine right away.

Different Patients, Different Treatments

People who enter treatment early in the course of their OUD and have suffered few consequences can do well on buprenorphine even without additional therapy. These individuals are usually emotionally mature to begin with, and they didn't use for long enough to destroy their lives. But teenagers or young adults, whose emotional maturity is stalled when they turn to drugs early on to cope with emotions, need help working through the surge of emotions and memories that erupt when they stop using opioids. Unwanted feelings create an edginess, a restless unease that can quickly drive people back to the warm solace given so freely by their drug of choice. These people benefit from learning new coping and social skills through therapy.

Buprenorphine is a ray of hope. It gives not only the person struggling with addiction but everyone in the family a chance to breathe and recuperate if even just a little from the ongoing chaos that swirls around a person with OUD. Family members go to bed without worrying about their loved one overdosing, for perhaps the first time in years. The addicted individual starts to feel somewhat normal, and their lack of craving for the drug does not go unnoticed. Everyone allows themselves some small permission to think that *maybe there is hope.*

I advocate that all patients with OUD be evaluated and, if appropriate, started on buprenorphine as soon as possible. Once they are on buprenorphine, the risk of overdose or other addiction-related consequences decreases dramatically. After that, they can undergo a thorough evaluation and all involved can decide the best approach to treatment long-term. It may be continuing with buprenorphine, transitioning onto methadone, or detoxification followed by a relapse prevention treatment with naltrexone.

After a patient is first prescribed buprenorphine, next steps depend on how they respond to the medication. Have cravings resolved enough to stop the desire to use? Are there side effects? Have their mood, sleep, energy, and appetite improved? The severity of the disorder, whether the patient has a coexisting medical or mental health condition, and whether they have a stable and supportive home environment are all factors that can affect treatment efforts. If any of these issues exist, addressing them is not optional. It is essential.

Later in this chapter, we will cover feasible treatment options, which might include finding a spot in a medication-based outpatient treatment clinic, where the patient receives ongoing therapy and can try naltrexone or methadone if buprenorphine is not doing the trick. But let's get past the first hurdle: Where do you go for buprenorphine?

Finding Help You Can Trust: Outlets for Buprenorphine

Access to buprenorphine is currently available in a limited number of settings, primarily in specialty addiction or mental health treatment programs. More and more family medical doctors, internists, and other nonspecialists, however, are being trained to offer buprenorphine. Once certified, nurse practitioners (NP), physician assistants (PA), and physicians (MD or DO) are able to prescribe buprenorphine. Dentists, pharmacists, and chiropractors cannot prescribe it.

Buprenorphine is a relatively safe medication. It does not require special monitoring beyond what is needed for other controlled substances prescribed by physicians. Treatment with buprenorphine can be implemented in almost any primary care setting. Knowing where you can get the medication in your community before you or your loved one is ready to seek help can make all the difference.

Family doctor: Like with any other condition, you can go to your family doctor. Call the community health center or private practice ahead of time and ask whether anyone is certified to prescribe buprenorphine. If yes, make an appointment to speak with the professional so you can discuss the situation, get feedback, and confirm that someone is able and ready to help when you need it. If none of your local clinics has such a provider, you can search a reputable internet database of certified providers, such as findtreatment.samhsa.gov. Once you find a name, call to confirm whether the provider is available. Some of the people listed are either no longer prescribing or have a wait list.

Many people with OUD prefer to be treated in a general clinic, where they do not feel stigmatized by being identified as "an addict." They sit in the waiting room among people with broken arms, diabetes, or heart disease. Ideally, someday, most patients with uncomplicated OUD will be able to seek treatment in a general health-care setting. However, if this is not available or appropriate for your loved one, ask to be referred to an addiction specialist.

Addiction specialist: An addiction specialist is a medical doctor, nurse practitioner, or a physician assistant with special training in addiction. Addiction specialists may practice alone. More commonly, they are part of a team at a specialized addition treatment program that may be licensed by the state to provide specialty treatment. If you have a referral, call the specialist and confirm that they are certified and available to prescribe buprenorphine. Ask them questions about how they work. Any program that provides treatment for OUD should offer medication, preferably buprenorphine and naltrexone. Opioid treatment programs primarily provide treatment with methadone, but some will also offer buprenorphine or naltrexone. If the program only offers "abstinence-based treatment," meaning they do not prescribe medications, look for another program. There is no evidence that treatment without medication is effective for OUD.

Professional organizations: Reach out to professional organizations that represent physicians to search for an addiction specialist in your area. This includes such organizations as the American Society of Addiction Medicine, American Academy of Addiction Psychiatry, American Osteopathic Academy of Addiction Medicine, and the American Psychiatric Association. These professional organizations list names and contact information for professionals trained in addiction medicine and psychiatry. Again, your first question should be, *Do you offer medical treatment for opioid use disorder?*

Health insurance companies: If you have health insurance, call and ask for a referral to an addiction specialist or a physician certified to provide treatment with buprenorphine. You may find that some of these doctors no longer offer this treatment or are not taking new patients, so brace yourself, because you may need to call many numbers.

Treatment on demand: As the name implies, treatment on demand (TOD) offers individuals with OUD immediate access to treatment. These clinics do not require an appointment. A person can walk in, be evaluated for opioid use disorder, and receive medication. TOD clinics are only beginning to pop up in the hardest-hit states. Some websites advertising "treatment on demand" are telemedicine sites that offer treatment over the internet using a video connection for patient-doctor meetings. As of the end of 2017, buprenorphine cannot be prescribed by a doctor who has not had at least one face-to-face meeting with the patient, and a video conference does not satisfy that requirement.

Traditional treatment points of entry often require a waiting period before medication is prescribed. This may be because the provider needs to complete a full evaluation, which takes time, or has reached a limit on the number of patients they can treat. When you call to make the appointment, ask when you can expect to start the medication. *Do not postpone starting buprenorphine because you have not found the ideal treatment setting.* If your loved one is on buprenorphine, you have the luxury of having some time to explore other treatment options.

Avoiding Treatment Traps

When most people start looking for treatment, they do one of two things: They call a friend, relative, or acquaintance who is in recovery and ask for advice, or they search the internet. With OUD, these logical approaches to finding help can backfire. Friends or relatives who've gone through a traditional abstinence-based program for alcoholism or a drug addiction may be doing well. They have good intentions in wanting to steer you toward traditional treatment. But if treatment without medication is their primary suggestion for your loved one, they are unwittingly putting your loved one in danger of experiencing an overdose during a relapse.

An internet search will yield many results. It also calls up advertising for websites that are set up as clearinghouses for treatment centers. Once these sites capture your information and your interest in seeking treatment, they sell it to the highest bidder—not necessarily to the best program. Some of these shady centers bidding for information don't really care whether their treatment fits the person's needs. They are looking for a body and insurance reimbursement. Desperate family members, vulnerable and prone to magical thinking, believe that this one decision to put their loved one in this center will change everything. They fall into a trap of believing empty promises.

When you break a leg, you go to an orthopedist. When dealing with addiction, you should seek the opinion of an addiction specialist. Know your options ahead of time, if at all possible. It will prevent your loved one from falling into the wrong hands. And you can move quickly when your loved one is ready.

Outpatient Versus Residential Treatment

Peoples are often disappointed when they learn their insurance may not cover residential treatment until they've "failed" outpatient. Residential programs have always been considered the gold standard of addiction treatment. But they may not necessarily be better for a person with OUD. While they offer their residents a lot in terms of services and supports, it is difficult to predict who will benefit from residential versus outpatient treatment. When treating OUD with medications, which requires long-term follow-up, outpatient treatment usually makes more sense financially and logistically.

Residential setting: In residential treatment, patients live at a treatment center usually for at least three to four weeks. They are first detoxified on the medical unit and then moved into the treatment setting with other patients, or they may receive a buprenorphine taper for a week while remaining in the general setting. They attend one-on-one counseling sessions and group therapy, get a full psychiatric evaluation, and have any necessary medications dispensed to them as needed. They receive education on the nature of addiction and the effects of drugs on their body, and they may receive evidence-based psychosocial or behavioral interventions, attend a family program, and work with assorted staff to implement a treatment plan. Upon discharge, they are given a relapse prevention plan, connected with their local recovery community, and referred to sober housing, if necessary. Residential treatment is the most intensive level of addiction care and is sometimes turned to after repeated relapses.

Residential treatment is an insulated setting. It is extremely difficult for patients to access their drug of choice, so it is nearly impossible to relapse while in residential treatment. Yet it is also expensive, costing somewhere in the neighborhood of $15,000 to $30,000 a month, and the price does not necessarily reflect the quality of treatment. Insurance or financial aid may cover a portion of it, but for most people, the cost is prohibitive. Residential programs do not refer to methadone maintenance and most do not offer buprenorphine except for a short time to alleviate withdrawal. A residential treatment program is an ideal setting to offer XR-naltrexone, as patients are fully detoxified and can receive it without concern about precipitating opioid withdrawal. Most residential programs, however, do not offer it.

Detoxed patients exiting residential centers that do not offer medication come out with some useful coping skills. But once back in the real world, these patients must be linked up with a physician who can prescribe medication. This can be a fairly smooth transition if it happens as soon as possible. In my experience, it is best to arrange for the patients to be transported directly from the residential program, with a family member or a trusted person, to the doctor's office to receive an XR-naltrexone injection or start buprenorphine if more appropriate. The residential center may or may not endorse this decision, so you may not be able to count on a referral or their support. But any delay in treatment puts these patients, who usually experience an increase in cravings upon returning home, at high risk of relapse. I have seen and heard too many painful stories of young adults relapsing and overdosing on the first or second day after leaving residential programs, before they had a chance to start outpatient treatment. Sadly, none of these patients was on medication to protect them against relapse.

Outpatient setting: Patients can enter various intensities of outpatient treatment. At a minimum, a patient visits the clinic once a month to get medicine and see a therapist once a week or less often. More intensive outpatient programs offer group therapy, usually two or three times per week, in addition to weekly individual therapy. The most intensive program is the day program, or what is known as a partial-hospital program. Patients go to treatment four to five days a week for four to five hours at a time. They are exposed to intensive evidence-based interventions and specialized treatment for medical or psychiatric diagnoses. When patients leave treatment at the end of the day, they have an opportunity to practice what they have learned in a real-world setting. The majority of outpatient programs do not offer buprenorphine or naltrexone, although this is gradually changing.

Treatment is like a circle. There is no real end. Individuals who complete a residential program may continue treatment for one to two months in a partial hospital and progress to a weekly outpatient program of gradually decreasing intensity, provided they continue to meet treatment goals. After six months or more, most patients may be fine with a monthly check-in. Because the best treatment is long-term treatment on medication, it is most important to find a good program that your loved one can stay in for months or years. You can spend $5,000 for one week at an out-of-state residential program or one month of local outpatient programming. I would choose the latter, provided that the program offers medications and evidence-based psychosocial interventions. Insurance may be more likely to cover the cost of outpatient treatment as well. Patients who remain actively involved in outpatient treatment in the long term are much more likely to do well than those who only complete a short-term intensive residential program, no matter how good the program is.

Because addiction is chronic, patients do well to be monitored. Increases in cravings, lapses to occasional use, or worsening of psychiatric problems are a call for more intense monitoring or treatment until the patient regains stability. This is the model of treatment most doctors use when managing patients with a serious mental illness such as recurrent depression, bipolar disorder, or schizophrenia.

No one should think they can ever fully graduate from treatment, as OUD cannot be cured with a treatment episode. People in recovery should be congratulated for staying in treatment, celebrate anniversaries for when their sobriety began, or applaud another year of having a good life while keeping OUD in remission.

A Program Scorecard

Outdated treatment efforts for OUD are at best a waste of time and money. At worst, they are downright harmful. If you know what to look

OUD Treatment Program Scorecard

You can compare treatment options using the program scorecard. In the scorecard, you are looking to fill in the "yes" column as much as possible. The first two services ("medication" and "medication taper not required") should always be marked "yes." You can fill this out over the phone. Just ask whether they offer each service. Not all of the services listed will be important to you or your loved one. Single out those you care about most.

Service	Yes	No
Medication (buprenorphine or naltrexone)		
Medication taper not required		
Interim treatment while on wait list		
Assessment of psychiatric and medical disorders		
Medical personnel (nurse, physician) on-site		
Psychiatrist on-site or available for consultation		
Licensed psychologist on-site		
Therapists adequately qualified		
Evidence-based therapies		
Cognitive behavioral therapy (CBT)		
Motivational enhancement therapy (MET)		
Contingency management (CM)		
Community reinforcement approach (CRA)		
Community reinforcement and family training (CRAFT)		
Behavioral couples therapy		
Strategic family therapy		
Multidimensional family therapy (MDFT)		
Acceptance and commitment therapy (ACT)		
Dialectical behavior therapy (DBT)		
Prolonged exposure therapy		
Mindfulness-based cognitive therapy		
Cognitive behavioral therapy for insomnia (CBT-I)		
Neuropsychological evaluation		
Nutritional counseling		
Physical and exercise counseling		

Service	Yes	No
Individualized treatment plan		
Individualized programming		
Flexible duration of treatment		
Group therapy		
Individual therapy		
Family program		
Treatment of co-occurring disorders with medication and therapy		
Coordination with a prescribing provider (if outside the program)		
Linkage to other evidence-based programs if additional treatment is needed		
Linkage to self-help groups in the community		
Recovery planning		

Other Questions to Ask Treatment Providers

- Do you prohibit the use of any medications? If yes, which medications?
- How long is the program?
- Is there a wait list?
- What does treatment cost?
- What are average out-of-pocket expenses after insurance?
- How do you help families use their health insurance to pay for treatment?
- What percentage of people are discharged on medications?
- What treatment do people usually go to after discharge?
- Do you follow up with people after they leave the program?
- Is there an option to follow up with the primary therapist on the phone after discharge? Is it a scheduled or "as-needed" follow-up?
- What happens if a person relapses and wants to come back to treatment?

for, you can avoid falling into a treatment trap. When looking for OUD treatment, the single most important factor is whether the facility offers evidence-based treatment that includes medication—buprenorphine or naltrexone. The second most important factor is having the option to stay on medication over the long term, without a predefined treatment duration. Some clinics approach medication as a temporary solution. They eventually require patients to decrease the amount of medication they are taking until they are medication-free, sometimes after only a few months. Stopping medications is never a goal when treating the most common chronic medical conditions, and it should not be a goal when treating OUD, which is the most lethal of all psychiatric disorders. Medications are well proven to decrease the risk of death. Although some people can eventually discontinue medication, it should not be required or even considered within the first few years of treatment.

Access to evidence-based treatment for addictions and co-occurring psychiatric disorders is an important consideration when selecting a treatment program. The qualifications of the therapists and medical providers supervising treatment are also worth asking about. Many addiction treatment programs employ counselors who are in recovery themselves but have little formal training in addiction. Some forms of therapy involve additional training and certification. Find out how much experience the therapist has and whether they receive supervision and ongoing training, which is important to maintaining a high quality of treatment.

A medical evaluation and treatment is best if it is offered by a physician, physician assistant, or nurse practitioner who is able to see your loved one regularly to monitor treatment efforts as well as possible side effects of the medication. Treatment is most effective if the physician can turn to all available medications, without restrictions. Some programs have a list of "prohibited medications" that usually include controlled substances, including buprenorphine. Preferably, staff members have training and experience working with people who have psychiatric disorders. Some programs may claim they treat co-occurring psychiatric disorders, but this may only include a one-time consultation with a psychiatrist. So, it is important to ask questions.

The best programs offer a comprehensive evaluation followed by a treatment plan individualized for each person, with a schedule of interventions and a description of treatment intensity and duration. Cost, insurance coverage, location, and other factors are important as well. But if the program does not offer evidence-based treatment, nothing else really matters. You will be setting your loved one up to fail.

Improving Access to Help

My goal, along with many others in my profession, is to see outlets for help expand soon and rapidly. If I had my way, each state or county would have a hotline, a dedicated phone number to call for help with opioid addiction that was posted on billboards and in bus stations, homeless shelters, unemployment lines, clinics, hospitals—anywhere and everywhere. You'd call the number and get the nearest location of a doctor certified to prescribe buprenorphine and taking patients, a program offering methadone, or an inpatient unit that can treat opioid withdrawal and start relapse prevention treatment with naltrexone. Anyone could start treatment the same or the next day, without considering ability to pay (financing long-term care would be approached later). All emergency rooms would offer buprenorphine on the spot to anyone who came in with an opioid overdose, a recent overdose, an injury related to opioid use, or just asking for help. There would be no wait lists, no confusion about where to go, no worries about whether you trust the people who say they can help you, no complicated instructions, and no concerns about what treatment would cost.

Once started on medication, patients would be referred to an addiction treatment program that offers a full evaluation and long-term treatment. Patients who do not need intensive treatment could get their medication and attend counseling and checkup appointments. The programs would also have team of professionals to help with the multitude of needs that other patients with addiction might present with: medical, psychiatric, educational, occupational, legal, family, childcare, transportation, housing, food, and other social needs. Each program would have access to peer supports (individuals themselves in recovery), to mutual-help communities, and to drug-free supportive housing. Each program would also have a community outreach arm that offers harm reduction interventions, including overdose prevention training, needle exchange, infection control education, and drug-testing services, as well as linkage to treatment.

In the nation's hardest-hit areas, treatment on demand and the comprehensive-care model outlined here are becoming more and more available. In northern Kentucky, for example, an active group of professional and grassroots activists is building programs of this kind. Their model could be made available everywhere and strongly supported by policy makers in each community.

OUD treatment should be available wherever you go for health care—the family doctor, the ER doctor, the pediatrician, the obstetrician, the psychiatrist. Health care is an established system. There's no reason not to align it with the medical model approach to treating OUD. Physicians do not need to be addiction experts to offer treatment to a large group of patients. They can conduct standardized screening and follow up with a brief in-person evaluation and a medical assessment. If the patient has OUD, they could prescribe buprenorphine and refer them to an addiction treatment center if such a program is available. If there is no program or if the wait list to get into the program is too long, the doctor could continue treating the patient as they do patients with any other chronic medical disorder.

The Family's Ongoing Role

Samantha (whose story is in chapter 8) had laid out a route for Eric that made it easy for him to get immediate help. She managed this because she had already done the legwork. She had talked to experts, gotten solid advice, and had names and numbers to call. She had consulted with Dr. Harrison and asked whether the doctor would go out of her way to see Eric when he was ready. Dr. Harrison was not an addiction expert, but she had taken the training required to administer buprenorphine. She also hadn't been living under a rock. She understood the tragedy of opioid addiction and knew that buprenorphine was a solid first line of defense. She wanted to be available to help in her community.

But Dr. Harrison's prescription wasn't the end of the road for Eric. It was just a beginning. Samantha and the rest of the family also had a long road before them. Not only did they need to heal from years of living with a person using heroin, they also had to make every effort to help Eric stay on track in his recovery.

CHAPTER 10

How to Support Your Loved One in Treatment and Recovery

I almost couldn't contain how happy I was," remembers Michael. He is referring to the road trip he took with his parents to treatment, one state and 160 miles from his home. "I knew recovery was going to be a long, hard journey. But I really wanted it. I really wanted recovery. Getting clean is easier to deal with if you really want it, and I couldn't wait."

During the drive to the rehab center, Michael's parents felt mostly relief. *Treatment will work*, they told themselves. For JoAnn, Michael's mom, failure was not an option. Treatment had to work. She knew she could not go through the experience again. Michael's parents had already lost all trust in Michael, who confers that "trust is lost in buckets but gained in drops." During the drive, he knew he would have to work hard to earn their trust again. And he wanted this just as much as he wanted to put his opioid use behind him.

Michael did all he could to make it in recovery. After a month in residential treatment, he went to a sober house for four months. He was drug tested daily, returned to his room a half hour before curfew without fail, and never broke a single rule. He attended an intensive outpatient program and asked to do the next level. His parents, encouraged yet apprehensive, told him "by all means."

At age twenty-three, Michael moved into a sober-living apartment in Manhattan with a recovering buddy. He knew the big city offered a lot in the way of temptation, but there was also a lot of recovery. Michael attended outpatient treatment five days a week, talked about his addiction at Twelve Step meetings, and saw a psychiatrist. Again, Michael's parents agreed to foot the bill but on one condition: Michael, who has an aversion to needles, had to get his monthly naltrexone injections. If he didn't show up, the doctor would let his parents know.

A year later, as Michael prepares to return to his hometown, he is overcome with anxiety. At home, triggers to use are everywhere. But Michael has an idea: There is a drug-testing lab three miles from his parents' home where he can get tested three times a week. His parents agree to pay for the testing.

After a year and a half on naltrexone, Michael feels solid enough in his recovery to stop taking the medication. He regularly attends Twelve Step meetings and sees a psychiatrist once a month. He doesn't have cravings, nor does he notice much of a difference, except on the twenty-eighth of each month, when he feels a phantom soreness, as if he had just gotten his monthly injection.

Michael is now taking classes to become an alcohol and drug counselor. Schools regularly invite him to speak to high school students about drug use, where he and his parents are told how impactful his speeches are.

Now that Michael has been sober four years, JoAnn has stopped picking apart the past to figure out what she did wrong as a parent. "It was like beating a dead horse," she says. "I was a stay-at-home mom, I knew where my kids were, I went to hockey games, volunteered in the school. I did the best that I could. I don't feel responsible for his drug use anymore."

While Michael's treatment cost a small fortune, JoAnn says it was worth every penny. And she is ever grateful the family had the resources. "When one door closes, another door opens. This horrible, horrible tragedy has opened up a whole new world to him where he can help people. For me, it was worth it. If he can get through to one kid, it will have been worth it."

Michael smiles when he talks about the dark days of using. He gets emotional, on the verge of tears, when he speaks of recovery. "There was a time when my parents didn't like talking about me," he says. "Now everyone is proud of me. Six months into my recovery, I was best man at my brother's wedding. When I was using, my brother wouldn't trust me to walk his dog. Now he lets me babysit his daughter. That might not sound like a big deal to some people, but to me, it's everything."

A New Beginning

Treatment does not signal the end of addiction. Addiction has no On and Off button. In time the brain heals, rerouting neuronal pathways as the recovering person practices new behaviors and creates new memories. But the genetic makeup and deeply learned behaviors connected to drug use still exist and will remain forever. Using can set off some of these pathways in an instant or after a matter of days or weeks. So, treatment is the beginning of recovery. It's a means to a new start—a chance to reinvent oneself or at least function without the constant longing for the powerful positive effects of opioids.

Michael's recovery sounds picture-perfect. At every juncture, his family backs him up, financially and emotionally. He stays in treatment as long as possible, takes his medication as prescribed, makes new friends, goes to self-help meetings, and goes back to school. With the support of his family, Michael creates a new, incredibly satisfying life for himself in recovery.

But even with everything going for Michael, he will tell you he didn't win the lottery. Recovery comes with trials and tribulations. It takes effort. Even when taking medicine, people can struggle in recovery, some more than others, especially during the first few months. The threat of relapse lingers, and triggers (of which there are many) can quickly turn into excuses to use again. Motivation level, quality of life, support system, and sense of personal responsibility are large factors in recovery. Preparation is also key—has the physician or addiction specialist informed their patients of what to expect and what to do if they feel that using is imminent? Is a prevention plan in place? Is there an emergency plan? Are family members involved?

Family members benefit from being prepared for what lies ahead. Thinking that everything will return to the way it used to be, before drug use, is self-deception. No one is the same, and life will be different. But different can also mean better.

Nicole's Recovery

Every month, Nicole goes to her appointment to get her naltrexone injection as if she were going to get her nails done. There is no drama, anxiety, mistrust, or arguments with family about keeping her appointments. Her medication works, and she is more than happy to take it. For Nicole, naltrexone blocks all thoughts of using.

Still, being opioid-free means emotions can hit Nicole when she least expects it. When her mom makes a casual comment about the dirty dishes in the sink, Nicole reacts. Her mom accuses her of being moody and jumps to the conclusion that Nicole is using again. But Nicole does not recall ever being defensive when using. She was checked out, just "there." In this argument, Nicole gets the last line: "I just feel more now, Mom. When I don't react—that's when you need to worry."

After seven months, Nicole reminds herself that she needs patience. She has every intention to stay in recovery and raise her son. But she knows that trust can take years to rebuild. She has lied, stolen, and been in and out of rehab for the past ten years. Her family is recovering, too.

Nicole is lucky. Although Jake, Robbie's father, is gone, and Nicole is a single parent, she has the unconditional love and support of her very large and close-knit family—and has had them all along. Even when Nicole was using, lying, and stealing, she felt loved and supported.

Robbie is doing exceptionally well. At age two, he has met all of his developmental milestones. He is healthy and happy, with a voracious appetite. Every day, he revels being in the company of more than one doting relative. And he adores his mom.

Nicole has just recently returned to work at her dad's contracting business. Working and raising a son leave her little time for much else. She does not attend Narcotics Anonymous or counseling. "The idea of sitting around talking about drugs made me want to use drugs. In my mind, it wasn't for me," she says. "I just want to live a normal life. Go to work, be with my family. Do normal things." For now at least, her family is support enough.

It doesn't occur to Nicole to stop getting her monthly naltrexone injections. It's not controlling her life or hurting her. As long as her insurance covers it, she can think of no reason to stop. Physically, mentally, and emotionally she feels better than ever.

For Nicole, recovery comes with pacifiers, sippy cups, and joyous giggles. "It's not just about me anymore. I have to keep reminding myself of that. Also, my son already has only one parent because of drug addiction. I want to live. I never did drugs because I wanted to die. I can't even tell you why I did drugs. I want to live and have a nice family.

"As hard as life can be sometimes, being in recovery is so much easier than using. Using makes everything so much harder."

Be an Asset in Recovery

You are likely well aware that you can't control addiction or the person in recovery, but you can be an asset. This is not to say that your loved one's recovery is your responsibility, but you and other family members play a large role. You influence whether recovery is easier or harder, a plus or a negative.

In early recovery, people need a lot of support, more than you might think necessary. Thinking and concentration can be foggy for a while, as the brain adjusts. Energy is low because a good night's sleep is hard to come by, at least initially. A car, job, or money might be issues. Basic skills, from hygiene to job interviewing, might be lacking. All of this is because of a serious chronic illness. If your loved one suffered from a serious disorder other than addiction, how would you treat them? Would you help them learn to do new things? Drive them to appointments? Support them financially? Make sure they take their medication? Help them apply for a job? Be forgiving?

Addiction gets a bad rap because addicted individuals hurt those they love. But if you think of addiction as a chronic disorder of the brain that impairs normal thought processes, it becomes easier to separate the disorder from the person. Although there is no cure for addiction, people can begin to heal the parts of the brain affected by ongoing drug use. Those who have support fare better than those who do not.

Everyone's experience is unique, yet we can predict events that can lead a person with opioid use disorder back to using. The number one deal breaker is not taking the medication—or taking too much.

Monitor Medications

Even the most motivated of patients can have a change of heart when it comes to taking their medication. Sometimes it is because the medication is working too well. About 50 percent of people stop taking buprenorphine after a while, and some do so because they feel they are back to "normal." Stopping medication because everything got much better happens even more often with XR-naltrexone, as there is no withdrawal or any other change right after naltrexone is stopped. Many people question whether they need to keep taking it, especially when they feel so good. Yet they still have a chronic disorder and are exposed to stress and cravings, which leave them vulnerable to relapse. Getting off medication can make maintaining abstinence much more challenging.

In one study, despite high levels of treatment satisfaction, more than 60 percent of patients maintained on buprenorphine or methadone expressed interest in discontinuing medication in the near future, and more than 70 percent had previously tried to stop—sometimes because of pressure from family or even the addiction professional being paid to help them. So, a major challenge is how to retain patients in treatment with medications and recovery over the long term. You can help by overseeing

Buprenorphine Misuse

It is possible to abuse buprenorphine. People will take more than the recommended dosage and run out before they can get a refill. They may take it because they still have cravings or to help with anxiety, stress, or depression. Buprenorphine is not meant to treat underlying psychiatric disorders, no matter how big the dose. In such cases, other psychiatric medications may be more helpful.

People can also get high on buprenorphine. They dissolve the strips and inject it to feel a positive, intoxicating effect that lasts several hours. Even the film and the tablet containing naloxone can produce euphoria if injected.

Patients may also decide to take less buprenorphine than prescribed or none at all for a few days. With no medication in the body to block a high, these individuals can use their drug of choice and feel effects. So taking less medications is also an issue.

It is important to monitor your loved one's supply of buprenorphine and store it in a safe place. When possible, make sure that every dose of buprenorphine is taken as prescribed, preferably all at once, first thing in the morning. If they complain that the dosage is not enough, listen and empathize and then encourage them to talk to their doctor and come up with a solution. The doctor may want to do "medication callbacks," whereby the doctor asks the patient to come to the office at random times with the leftover medication to make sure it is being taken as prescribed. A long-acting buprenorphine injection may be a good solution for patients who have difficulty taking daily doses of buprenorphine as prescribed.

the medication and making sure your loved one takes it on schedule. Michael's parents, for instance, set this condition: If Michael didn't show up for his naltrexone injection appointments, they would stop paying for his treatment and his apartment.

I find that the adolescents and young adults whose parents are closely involved in monitoring the medication tend to do better than those with less oversight. These parents come to each appointment, give an update, witness the naltrexone injection, and ask how they can be involved. Patients eighteen and older need to give permission to keep the communication open, but many want to do so once they see the benefits. Others give their parents access to the results of drug screens as a condition of receiving continuing support. The same happens with older adults who bring their spouse or significant other and make them an active participant in treatment. Some people are involved for a while or only if something bad happens. Or they stay involved for a year or two. For patients doing well in recovery, the gradual transition away from involving significant others in treatment can work. The independence translates as trust, and this is progress. Eventually, everyone must become personally responsible for their own recovery.

How you can help:
- Be present when the medication is picked up from the pharmacy.
- Help keep medication in a safe place.
- Dispense it at scheduled times or in small amounts.
- Supervise when medication is taken.
- Accompany your loved one for naltrexone or buprenorphine injections or implantation surgery.
- Set clear expectations for taking medication.
- Clearly communicate benefits and rewards for taking medication and consequences for not taking it.

Accept Ambivalence as Part of Recovery

Ambivalence about being in recovery is one reason people don't take their medication or go to counseling. On days when your loved one feels stressed or low, the numbing or uplifting effect of opioids might sound attractive. When bored, your loved one might recall some of the good times they had with their using friends. These kinds of thoughts can put a recovering person in a using frame of mind. They might act and sound as if recovery is not for them and a waste of time. On other days, they are happy and grateful to wake up without wondering how to get their next fix. They are elated to know that they have a job to go to or a child to cuddle.

Ambivalence is normal. People in the grip of addiction look for reasons to use. Sometimes your loved one will be motivated for abstinence; other days they will feel conflicted. Once you expect and accept this, you will find the seesaw characteristics of ambivalence much easier to deal with.

We do not berate soon-to-be brides or grooms for questioning the decision to marry. We listen, comfort, and try to understand what they are thinking or feeling. We accept it as a normal part of the process, because marriage is a big commitment with lots of unknowns. The same is true with recovery. Giving up the freedom to use is a commitment. Your loved one grieves their loss at the same time that they are learning to participate in life again. When participating in life gets hard or dull, ambivalence grows.

It's also important to validate that there are downsides to abstinence, at least initially. Be open to seeing recovery challenges from your loved one's perspective.

How you can help:
- Ask questions to learn why your loved one is feeling unsure.
- Ask about their reasons for change and their belief in the ability to change.
- Emphasize their strengths, all the positive actions they have already taken.
- Create a contingency plan for when cravings are strong, one that you can be involved in.

The Importance of a Contingency Management Plan

A contingency management plan (CMT) is a written "contract" you can use to reward behaviors that are good for recovery and discourage behaviors that are not good for recovery. A CMT establishes expectations, sets limits, and outlines consequences. Guidelines and consequences are stated clearly and deliberately. Everyone in the household knows what is expected of them.

Ideally, all family members negotiate the CMT, and everyone agrees with the final decisions. You will want to review the plan with the treatment clinic or physician you are working with, as they will likely have good suggestions. But here are some ideas to get you started:

- You can live in the house provided you respect house rules and respect all who live there.
- You agree to take your medicine in front of us and go to all doctor and therapy appointments.
- You agree to give your doctor permission to let us know when you miss an appointment or when your drug test shows recent use. If this happens, we will come to the appointment together to review the plan.
- If you take your medication, go to your appointments, and otherwise do your part, we will not bring up your past behavior and will provide food and housing.
- We will drive you to all your appointments and meetings, and we will pay for the medication and doctor's visits, but you must look for a job to help pay for gas.
- You agree that you will not cash your paycheck or hold large amounts of money, as this has been a big trigger for drug use in the past.
- If you start using regularly, you may still live in the house under the same rules, but you will need to pay for food.

- Suggest interesting activities that all family members can participate in.
- Encourage and actively support participation in self-help groups.

When a Family Member Is Opposed to Medication

A detrimental yet all-too-common mistake is when family members try to convince their spouse or child or parent to stop taking OUD medication. The notion that a person in recovery should not take medication is frustratingly common among family members. This mind-set usually stems from stigma or misunderstanding about the nature of OUD. People do not fully comprehend what it takes to recover from the disorder. Family members who would not question why their spouse needs to take medication many years after a cancer goes into remission should not question the need to take medication to prevent addiction from recurring. The focus on taking medication, rather than on recovery itself, creates turmoil and gets some patients and families into trouble. For Eric, it created a reason to think about using again.

Although Eric feels good on buprenorphine and Samantha is more than happy that her son is no longer shooting up heroin, Tom, Eric's dad, is sullen. He distances himself from Eric and his "recovery." If he thinks about it too much, Tom gets angry. His son has caused enough grief and wasted enough family resources already. He wants to put Eric's addiction behind him. He wants his son to buck up and face life without any drugs—including his buprenorphine, which Tom thinks is a crutch or just another way to get high. Although Samantha tries to stay matter-of-fact when Tom brings up Eric's medication, Tom and Samantha argue. Hearing the fights, and knowing he is the cause, brings Eric to the verge of tears. His guilt over not being able to stay abstinent in college and his remorse over failing his family, mixed with the good feelings he has taking buprenorphine, leave him feeling confused.

Eric considers that maybe his dad is right. Maybe it is better to recover without meds. It has been two months, he has not used once, and maybe he is ready.

Samantha has been keeping a close eye on Eric, making sure he takes his medicine in front of her every day. This is one of the family rules, and Eric is fine with it. He feels a little like a kid, yet he is grateful. But this evening, he tells his mom he is going out for an early morning run and not to bother getting up early. He promises to take his medication.

Eric goes for a run. He takes a tablet from the bottle but flushes it down the toilet. He feels pretty good for the rest of the day, and his mom believes Eric has followed through with his promise. That evening, Eric goes to work. A co-worker comes in high, and Eric starts having thoughts about using for the first time in two months. He snorts a small bit of heroin and feels great. He is not high enough to feel intoxicated but remembers how much he enjoyed the blissful effect. The next morning, Eric wakes up and Samantha dispenses his medication.

In one short evening, Eric has learned that he can play the game of skipping his medication so he can get high every now and then. His early-morning runs are a great cover-up. On those days, Eric goes to work and snorts a little, but the third time he does this he starts thinking of what it feels like to inject heroin. He stays out all night, without calling or letting his parents know that he has plans.

Eric has broken a major house rule. Samantha is convinced Eric has lapsed. Before confronting Eric, Samantha shares her suspicion with Tom and the psychiatrist. Tom is no longer angry but concerned. He thinks Eric has lapsed, too. Eric was doing well, and Tom didn't see this coming. The psychiatrist makes it clear that Tom and Samantha need to be allies in this battle. Tom agrees. That morning, they confront Eric in unison, and he caves in.

Ambivalence feeds on discord, and the person who is still hostage to addictive thinking may eventually fall prey to it. Family members who are pitted against one another need to talk and agree on a plan. Base your plan on the best evidence-based treatment and seek input from a professional. The family member who is skeptical about medication should speak with the doctor directly. Families must present a unified front toward the affected family member. There is no way around it. Families who do not agree about how to handle recovery can be torn apart by this type of thing.

Do your best to focus on what matters. What is your loved one's life becoming? If they are happier and involved in activities, it should not matter whether they take an antipsychotic, antihypertension, or antiaddiction medication. The objective is to improve and stabilize their life. Coming off medication should never be on top of the list. It can be low on the list, if it is on the list at all. Stigma around taking medicine and false expectations about recovery are leading causes of relapse.

How you can help:
- Insist on meeting with the doctor and the therapist.
- Know the treatment plan.
- Have a contingency plan if the current plan fails.
- Learn why your loved one was prescribed the medication they are taking.
- Learn all you can about this medication so you can support its use.
- Make sure everyone in the family agrees and supports the plan.
- Ask how you can be involved.

How you can help family members who struggle with accepting medications for their loved one:
- Validate their concerns and feelings.
- Try to understand where the belief is coming from (anger, hurt, disappointment).
- Keep them involved and informed—share how your loved one is improving on medication.

- Act as if they are interested by treating them as someone who wants to be updated—that is, stay in touch even if you have a difference of opinion.
- Avoid being pushy or angry.
- Encourage them to talk to the doctor.

Myths About Medication and Recovery

- You cannot be truly sober and in recovery if you take medication to help you quit using
- Medication gets in the way of your recovery work

When the Person in Recovery Wants to Discontinue Medication

George used to see his psychiatrist once a month, then every two months. Now, after three years on buprenorphine, he goes four to five times a year, mostly to talk about major events in his life and what might be stressing him out. He knows that uncomfortable and unaddressed feelings, or getting on a wrong train of thought, can lead him back to pills. George has considered getting off buprenorphine but cannot find a good enough reason to. It works for him, and he has already tapered down to 2 milligrams a day. His wife, who at first questioned the need for staying on medication that long, has fully accepted the idea. She sees that it works, and she has her husband back.

When patients tell me they want to stop using their medication, I keep an open mind. Some patients do indeed seem ready. They are on a low dose, have a solid support system, have a stable job they love, and seem to enjoy the benefits of therapy. They are motivated and have found ways to better fill the time they once spent finding and using drugs. They have a lot of what we call "recovery capital," enough positives in their lives to

Accumulating "Recovery Capital"

People in recovery earn what we sometimes call "recovery capital," or a buildup of positives in life. These are the assets that people collect slowly along the way by making thoughtful decisions in their lives. Recovery capital helps you stay in recovery. It is like money in the bank. On good days, you add to your savings. On a rainy day, or those times when you struggle, you can draw from it. The best way to build recovery capital is to keep it in mind at all times and work on accumulating it over a long time. Some of those assets include:

- Participate in treatment and continuing care
- Take advantage of therapy even if you have been doing well for a long time
- Actively engage with a mutual self-help community
- Take antiaddiction medication (buprenorphine, methadone, naltrexone) and any other medication your doctor recommends
- Find a primary care doctor, regularly go for checkups, and follow all recommendations to take good care of your physical health
- Eat regular nutritious meals and exercise regularly
- Seek and nurture friends who support your recovery
- Encourage your partner and family to support your recovery
- Find a community you can be a part of, whether religious, political, or people you share common interests with
- Actively contribute to the community you live in; be of service to others
- Support others in their recovery
- Choose to live in an environment that is free of drugs
- Make sure your home is secure and in a safe neighborhood
- Finish your education; find a stable and fulfilling job
- Clear all your past legal problems

help carry them through the more difficult days. Others have little in the way of recovery capital but begin to feel like their old selves again, which makes medication seem no longer necessary.

All patients need to understand the risks of tapering off medication. After discussing the pros and cons with patients who are ready (that is, who have plenty of recovery capital), the doctor can taper, or slowly wean, them off the medication, and monitor how they are doing. Some patients reach a stage during the taper where cravings, discomfort, and agitation get to be too much, which is what happened with George. Not being able to taper off completely is not failure by any means, although patients sometimes feel this way. Most decide they are fine staying on the medication at a low dose.

Life does not stand still for someone because they are in recovery, and so I recommend ongoing counseling whenever possible. If a stressful situation presents itself, people may need to return to medication or increase their dosage, at least temporarily. Sometimes, a conversation with a therapist is medicine enough.

How you can help:
- Encourage a focus on recovery, not medication, but be open to thoughts about tapering.
- Ask your loved one why they want to stop medication.
- Talk about how confident they are in their recovery and how they will deal with craving and stress if these return once off medication.
- Insist that they speak with the doctor about whether they are ready.
- Go to the appointment with your loved one and ask to be involved.

Support Attendance at Appointments and Meetings

Psychological and behavioral treatments as part of ongoing counseling or outpatient treatment give professionals an opportunity to assess the progress of people in recovery. They can talk through stressful situations or identify disruptive thoughts and behaviors that can lead to drug use.

Such groups as Narcotics Anonymous (NA) help people understand they are not alone. Others like them have gone through some of the same experiences and come out stronger. NA welcomes people who are on medication to attend meetings, but not all members will see attendees who are taking medicine as being abstinent, or in recovery. Do not force your loved one to go to meetings, but if they are interested in doing so, support them.

How you can help:
- Schedule appointments for dentists, doctors, counseling.
- Find mutual-help meetings.
- Drive your loved one to appointments and meetings.
- Loan your car.
- Help decipher the bus or train schedule.
- Pay for a cab ride.

Encourage Abstinence

Abstinence is a troublesome word when discussing medication-assisted treatment. Because buprenorphine and methadone are opioids, they are considered mood altering, yet they are not the same as other opioids. Taking painkillers and heroin is considered "using." Taking methadone or buprenorphine as prescribed should not produce any immediate effect on the mood, is not intoxicating, and therefore does not contradict the idea of recovery. The same applies to other psychiatric medications, such antidepressants, antipsychotics, or mood stabilizers, which can of course "alter mood." Some psychiatric medications that are controlled substances, such as antianxiety or sleep medications or medications to treat ADHD, are also occasionally considered to be "off-limits" for a recovering person. This notion is based on the same assumption that considers buprenorphine, another controlled substance, inconsistent with recovery. If used properly, any of the medications used to treat underlying psychiatric symptoms can only help rather than impair recovery. An untreated psychiatric symptom is one of the top reasons for relapse. Occasionally, psychiatric medications are misused or have more side effects than benefits, but for the most part they are effective if given under close monitoring by an experienced addiction specialist. If people take medications, including controlled substances, but do not use any other mood-altering drugs, they are still sober. This is the new definition of recovery, despite what some people believe.

For the brain to fully heal, a long period of abstinence is necessary. Staying away from all mood-altering drugs, even alcohol, promotes recovery. On medication, staying away from opioids becomes easier. But if your loved one starts feeling "normal," pouring a drink or grabbing a beer might seem like a good idea to them. People with addiction can easily justify that some drugs are not a problem for them. And the intoxicating effects of any drug can weaken resolve. Under the influence, your loved one could decide that using opioids is not such a bad idea after all. And while it may be true that some will be able to use another drug recreationally and not get addicted, there is no way to predict who will be able to do so. In my opinion, the risk of "getting it wrong" is too high and not justified, definitely not in the first one to two years of recovery.

Everyone in the family has to review their relationship with drugs and put their use on hold. Drinking or smoking weed in front of the person in early recovery is a trigger. Having painkillers around is detrimental. In time, your loved one may not see alcohol as a trigger.

How you can help:
- Remove all drug paraphernalia from the home.
- Remove all alcohol and other drugs from the home.
- If you are prescribed painkillers, lock them up and do not take them in front of your loved one.
- Avoid using all other drugs, including alcohol, in front of your loved one; set a new normal—a drug-free home.
- Understand that early on your loved one must miss parties where alcohol or other drugs may be present.

Stay in the Solution

The solution for how to manage life with OUD is recovery. So do what you can to make recovery attractive. Being nagged about not exercising is an excuse to use, whereas being offered a membership to or ride to the gym or a yoga class is affirming, supportive, and positive. When being in recovery is more attractive than using, staying in recovery is easier and more likely.

Relapse is about what is happening inside as well as outside of the person in recovery—their feelings, thoughts, and environment. If they are bored or hanging out with using friends, identify the problem and help them think of the solution. Help them find new activities to stay busy and engaged; invite them to new places where they might have a good time and meet new friends. Do what you can to eliminate barriers and avoid the temptation to point fingers. Do what you can to encourage your loved one to want to be on the recovery side of the fence.

Being involved and positive enables recovery, which is a good thing. This high level of involvement is not lifelong. In time, your loved one will be more self-motivated and will eventually reciprocate. Positive behavior is contagious.

How you can help:
- Be positive and resourceful.
- Stay in the solution.
- Reinforce positive behaviors.
- Praise strengths.
- Try to see things from their perspective.
- Be grateful.

When Relapse Happens

Some people really struggle in recovery and may relapse one or more times before they find it. Others decide to give up before they even give recovery a chance because it is too hard. Environment, mental health, physical health, financial stability, friends and family, and the level of motivation and denial are only a few of the many factors that merge to either lift people up or drag them down during recovery. When the barriers people must surmount seem too great, and the urge to use is more powerful than the desire to get better, people may relapse.

Relapse is heartbreaking, yet it is a normal part of the process for many opioid users, some of whom relapse multiple times, especially if they do not have a chance to try medication. Opioids are powerful drugs, and the craving for them can be even more powerful. Medication can minimize or eliminate relapse and improve quality of life in most patients, but it is not failure proof. Doctors may need to adjust your loved one's medication dosage or change medications. Patients may need to take medications for depression or PTSD and add therapy to their treatment regimen.

The suggestions outlined in this chapter give you some tools to encourage your loved one to stick with recovery and recognize when something is awry. If relapse does occur, make sure your loved one returns to treatment as soon as possible. You can repeat what you did in the first place to get them to treatment.

OUD is a serious disorder. Relapse does not mean that the treatment was not impactful; it only means that it was not sufficient at that time and that it needs to be repeated. Intensity of treatment should match the severity of the disorder. When symptoms recur, the treatment needs to be repeated and possibly upgraded. This is the same standard used to treat most chronic medical disorders. Some patients may need to stay in treatment and on medications for the rest of their lives to get the disorder fully under control. We are fortunate to have medications to treat OUD. To this day, we do not have effective treatment for a number of serious and debilitating disorders.

Everyone Is in Recovery

Recovery is a time to exhale, but not fully. As your loved one adjusts to new feelings and the new way in which they must now operate in the world, you and other family members need to shift gears and recalculate where you stand. You will have a new role in the new family dynamic, which changes how you interact with your loved one. You will also need to rediscover the parts of your life that you have disconnected from—the friends, hobbies, and interests you dropped to focus on the addiction. In other words, you will be recovering, too.

Recovery is not intuitive. It is hard to see how another's addiction changes and reshapes us. I always recommend involving the family in the recovery. Recovery is not guaranteed. Relapse is forever a possibility. Therapy teaches people how to live with the uncertainty inherent in recovery. Therapy helps people see what has happened to their sense of self, as well as how their behaviors affect their loved one's recovery.

When efforts at recovery fail repeatedly, you need to protect your sanity. Counseling helped Lacey draw some desperately needed boundaries for herself when Jason's third attempt at treatment did not go well.

Lacey's New Boundaries

Shortly before Jason's third treatment, and against his wishes, Lacey started therapy for herself. Jason berated her with such lines as, "It's too expensive" or, "You don't have time for this" or, "I need you here to help me." But because of therapy, Lacey feels stronger. She stands her ground and keeps going.

When Jason enters residential treatment, Lacey attends the family program. Livid at Jason, she does not absorb all of what she is offered in the way of tools and supports. Still, she is grateful. She learns a lot about the dynamics of addiction and identifies with other spouses who are in the same boat. A woman in treatment for alcoholism for the tenth time attends Lacey's small-group session. She shares that in the past she went to treatment for her husband. This time, she is going for herself, and she is hopeful. This rings true with Lacey, who cringes at the thought of Jason's claiming to be in treatment for her and their daughters.

Lacey also goes to Al-Anon, the Twelve Step support group for spouses of people struggling with addiction and alcoholism. She at first searches for out-of-town meetings, where she will not run into anyone she knows, but the travel time is a constraint. Finally, she breaks down and goes to the meeting nearest her home. Glancing around the room, she sees four people she knows, but she does not care. Hiding the addiction and the family "shame" is suddenly no longer a priority. She has reached her limit, the place where enough is enough. She is done pretending and feeling crazy.

In Al-Anon, Lacey learns that she is not crazy. The people around her tell stories that are both disturbingly and refreshingly similar to hers—if not in the details, in the emotions. She begins to realize what has been happening to her. She is awash in relief and regret as she remembers who she used to be and considers the empty, angry shell of a person she has become.

Before Jason comes home from treatment, Lacey "is done." She can't seem to find any other words. She is done with the lies, the manipulation, the self-pity, and the excuses. When Jason comes home after twenty-eight days and against his treatment team's recommendations, he is faced with a more confident Lacey, who for the first time feels sure of herself in creating boundaries and consequences. He learns that if he uses, she will file for divorce. Two weeks later, when he overmedicates, drops food all over himself and the floor, and starts asking where his handgun is before he overdoses—all in front of her parents—Lacey not only calls the police but files for a divorce.

Lacey has turned the TV on maybe four times in the four months since she kicked Jason out of the house. After having it on 24/7, the sound of voices and assorted noises emanating from the box is now a source of trauma for her. Her youngest daughter is away at college, getting straight A's after having initially flunked out. Her thoughts are now focused on her studies, rather than worrying about whether her mom is okay. Lacey and her daughters continue to get therapy, which she says has made a world of difference.

PART 4

For Patients: What to Expect in Treatment and Beyond

CHAPTER 11

Getting Ready to Stop Using Opioids

It may be scary to think about the first days and weeks without your drug. This is normal. All people addicted to opioids stiffen up if they think about withdrawal. Many people keep using just to avoid withdrawal. But going through complete withdrawal is not always necessary. Some of the treatments available today do not require detoxification.

For most people, giving up drugs is a big decision. It is a major life change. The key to success in treatment is to be prepared. Having a good plan to follow helps you know what to expect so you are not surprised. A good plan starts with understanding yourself and the decision you are about to make.

The better you know yourself, the easier it will be for you to make this change. A good way to understand yourself and why you use is to ask yourself some questions. If you are not working with a therapist, you can do this on your own. It may be even better to do it with someone who knows you well and is supportive. I suggest that you do not begin treatment until you spend some time understanding yourself and your situation.

Understanding Your Strengths

Everyone has problems. Everyone also has the ability to overcome many of them. The first step to understanding your situation is to know what your problems are—as well as your strengths. When you were using, you had to be resourceful. You can use some of those same skills in positive ways to solve some of your problems.

Fill in the blanks in the chart. The first column lists different aspects of your life. You can add to this column, if you want. The second column is blank. Here, list one or two problems you have in this area of your life. In column three, list your strengths, or some of the skills you possess that can help you solve or deal with your problem. These are resources you can use as you embark on the journey toward a drug-free and fulfilling life.

Your Problems and Strengths

	My Problem	My Strengths & Resources
Health		
Mental Health		
Relationships with Family		
Relationships with Friends		

Your Problems and Strengths

	My Problem	My Strengths & Resources
Housing		
Employment		
Finances		
Community		
Spiritual Life		

Understanding Your Hopes

Now think about your hopes and aspirations. When you started using drugs regularly, you might have given up a lot of your interests. Allow yourself to think about the positive things that can be a part of your life. When you stop using drugs, you will likely have a lot of free time and extra money. Most people don't expect this. You may want to plan what you will do with that time.

Think about fun activities, like taking trips you always wanted to go on. Write them down. Next, write down some things that are good for you long-term, such as training for a new job. Imagine yourself three to six months from now. What will you be doing, where will you be living, who will be in your life, and how you will be spending your free time? Then imagine yourself in two to three years. Ask yourself the same questions.

Write down your answers. Exercises like this help you understand your thoughts and feelings more clearly. Writing things down improves mental health. Later, you can go back to what you wrote and see how far you have come.

Understanding Why You Use

An important part of getting ready to stop using is to think about why you take opioids. You might have been using opioids for a while, and you may not remember why you started in the first place. You probably took them because it felt really good to get high. But often there are other reasons for taking drugs. Many people use opioids because it helps them deal with chronic physical pain, emotional pain, bad memories, or daily stress.

You likely have other reasons for continuing to use. You may feel as if the only reason you take opioids now is to stop yourself from getting sick, but there is usually more to it. People keep using opioids because they are able to get high, even though the high is not the same as it was at first. They also keep using because they cannot imagine not using, or fear having to face life without their drug of choice.

The more you think about your reasons for using, the better you will be able to deal with difficult situations that come up. Try to think about those reasons. Make a list.

Look at your list. What will change when you stop using? Will you need to change anything else? Are you prepared to manage these changes? If using helps you forget about your problems, what will happen to these problems when you stop using?

The goal of this self-exploration is to help you see why you are in your situation. If you can see your situation more clearly, it is easier to change it.

Understanding the Decision to Stop Taking Drugs

Almost everyone who decides to stop using drugs is conflicted about this decision. The same may be true for you. Part of you really wants to change. You want to feel better and want problems to go away. But another part of you does not want to give up the option of using drugs. You may find them useful or fun. Those two voices are in a constant conflict, because only one can be right at any given time.

One of these two voices will be more or less dominant at first. There is nothing wrong with this; it is the nature of the struggle with drug addiction. It is best to recognize and accept it. Observe how your mind works rather than trying to suppress or avoid those thoughts. As you progress through treatment, you will notice that your thinking will also begin to change. Your voice for change will become stronger. But you will also go through difficult moments when the voice against change is stronger. This is normal.

Before you begin the journey, allow yourself to explore these two voices. Again, it is useful to write your thoughts down and go back to the list as you go through treatment.

Conflicting Voices

	Good things about it	Bad things about it
Quit using		
Continue using		

Here are a few suggestions for your list, but try to think of some that are your own:

- Being healthier
- Being happier
- Having more money
- Being safer, less risk of overdose
- Staying out of legal trouble
- Having energy and freedom to do stuff
- Getting to try new things
- Having options to deal with stress
- Fewer conflicts at home
- Fewer problems at work

- Going back to school or getting a job
- Going through withdrawal
- Missing fun and excitement
- Boredom
- Missing drug buddies

Alternatives to Coming off Opioids

Having gone through the first few exercises, you may decide that you are not yet ready to stop using. Many people are not ready to give up opioids. If you decide for now to keep using, you can still make some changes to help you stay safe.

Many cities and states have organizations committed to protecting the rights and health of people who use drugs. Examples of these groups are the Harm Reduction Coalition and the Drug Policy Alliance. They can tell you what services are available in your community for people who use drugs. You can learn where to exchange dirty needles for clean needles, get overdose kits, or get tested for HIV/AIDS. Some of them offer free counseling and support. They are there to help you stay safe, in the hope that one day you will decide to quit using. If you decide to quit using, these groups can quickly connect you to treatment. If you live near a harm reduction center, you should definitely check it out.

Meanwhile, consider the following:
- *Do not mix drugs.* This is the number one reason people overdose. Do not take alcohol or sedatives and opioids on the same day.
- *Know what you are using.* Get your drugs tested at a harm reduction center to make sure you know what you are taking. You may unknowingly buy heroin pills laced with dangerous substances. They will not get you high and may have really bad effects.
- *Use safely.* Try to stop injecting. Sniffing or smoking is safer. If you must inject, try to do it less often. Always use new needles. If you do not have any, use a disinfecting kit. Finally, never share needles and always use condoms when you have sex.

- *Keep naloxone nearby.* If you overdose, a witness can give you the overdose antidote.

You can also start addressing health and life problems. Visit a doctor if you have illness or pain. Go to social services to see about health insurance, housing, or food stamps. See whether you can reconnect with your family or friends who do not use drugs and let them know that you are thinking about stopping drugs. Try going to a local Narcotics Anonymous meeting. Let them know that you are thinking about stopping and see whether they have any good advice.

Knowing what happens in treatment might help you in your decision to quit using. Some treatment centers have peer advocates or navigators. These are people who are in treatment. They show you around and answer questions.

Many people are at first scared of the treatment experience. Many of these same people also come to thoroughly enjoy their new lives in recovery. Learn more about treatment even if you are not ready to stop using now.

Let's look at what you can expect in treatment.

Treatment

The three main treatment options for opioid use disorder

Taking medication to transition away from your opioid of choice into a life in recovery is proven to be the most effective treatment. In rare cases, it may be appropriate to transition into treatment that does not offer medication. But using medication is the safest route. Each medication works differently, but all of them make it easier for you to begin the journey into recovery.

You can stop using painkillers or heroin with the help of one of three medications:

- Methadone
- Buprenorphine

- Naltrexone

If the medication you start with does not work for you, you continue to have cravings, or you do not feel well, you can try a different one. If you find one that works well for you, you can stay on it for as long as you need to. Many people stay on medication for the rest of their lives. They are happy they found a medication that makes their lives so much better without the use of illicit opioids.

Who can help

You will want to find a treatment provider who offers safe and effective treatment for people addicted to opioids. The provider should be able to offer you buprenorphine or naltrexone, or they should be willing to send you to a methadone clinic.

A medical provider who treats opioid addiction can guide you through the treatment process. This can be a physician (MD or DO), a nurse practitioner (NP), or a physician assistant (PA). All of these providers can prescribe medications that will alleviate some of the withdrawal symptoms. They can also prescribe medication to help prevent relapse. These providers can supervise your treatment to make sure it is safe and successful. Or they can refer you to someone who can help.

Do not try treatment by getting medication from friends who are on the medication. It may sound like a good idea, but you may run into trouble while starting it or down the road. I have heard too many stories of patients who first tried to take medication from their friends, had a bad experience, and later were hesitant to try that medication again with a doctor.

No Medication Is Perfect

Medication for opioid use disorder is not a cure-all. Medication helps you stay abstinent so you can focus on recovery work. It also can save your life by preventing relapse and overdose. But it might not completely eliminate discomfort and craving, at least not in the beginning. And your life probably won't change for the better overnight. Many life changes will take effort on your part. Regardless of which route you choose, you will experience some uncomfortable thoughts and feelings within the first days and weeks. Being prepared for it can make all the difference.

If you take one of the medications, you might experience some side effects. The medications are designed to help with craving, withdrawal, and to prevent relapse. Relapsing is still a possibility, but medication is your best chance at recovery.

If you can deal with the life of a person addicted to opioids, you can probably deal with the discomforts of early recovery. After a while, your life will likely be much better than it was in the last months of your active addiction.

So your first big decision is whether you want to avoid detox at first and start your treatment using opioid-like medications or go through withdrawal and then use medication to prevent relapse. Let's look at each of the medications more closely.

Methadone

Methadone is an opioid, but when it is given as a medication, the body responds to it differently than it does to heroin and other opioids. On methadone, you will not feel intoxicated or in withdrawal. You will feel closer to "normal," or stable all the time.

Methadone is the mildest way to come off high doses of heroin or other opioids. You do not need to be detoxed before you start methadone. You will continue to be physically dependent on methadone and have to take it every day to avoid withdrawal. Think of it as a small price to pay for getting your life back.

Methadone may also discourage you from using your opioid of choice. Methadone blocks the high you would normally get from heroin or painkillers. Just knowing that helps many people stay abstinent.

Methadone is the most effective medication for treating opioid use disorder. It is also a powerful medication with possible side effects. If you take too much of it, or combine it with other sedatives, you can overdose.

Because of that risk, dosing of methadone has to be supervised at the clinic until you become used to it and your addiction is under control.

Like any medication, methadone has its pros and cons.

Pros: If you are on methadone, you will:
- Avoid overdose and death
- Avoid going into withdrawal
- Stop obsessing about finding drugs
- Avoid medical problems
- Spend less money
- Avoid jail or prison
- Take an opioid once a day by mouth and feel fine
- Find it is helpful as long as you keep taking it
- Have access to therapy and many services that your methadone program offers

Cons: Some of the downsides to using methadone are that you:
- Have to find a clinic that is taking new patients
- Must apply to get into a clinic and approval can take a few days or weeks
- Won't get high on it if taken as prescribed and will not be able to get high on opioids
- Have to take it every day or you will start going into withdrawal
- Have to go to the methadone clinic almost every day in the beginning
- May have side effects
- Can overdose if you take too much of methadone or take it in combination with sedatives, or if you stop taking methadone and relapse to heroin use

If you start methadone, your first job is to take the medication every day as prescribed, participate in therapy sessions, and not take any other opioids. If you continue to have urges to use, ask for a dose increase.

Higher doses are more helpful than lower doses. If you can stay with daily methadone and not use any other opioids, other drugs, or alcohol, you are doing well.

Once you are able to stay abstinent from illicit opioids for about three months, you may start getting doses to take home, so that you do not have to come to clinic every day. Over time, as long as you stay abstinent and make progress, you may need to come to the clinic only once per week.

Some people stay on methadone for years and do very well. Other people transition to buprenorphine.

Buprenorphine

Buprenorphine is a weak opioid. It allows you to feel some of the effects of opioids but less than you would get if taking methadone. Otherwise, buprenorphine works the same as methadone. Buprenorphine reduces the craving for your drug of choice. It also minimizes other withdrawal symptoms. You do not need to go through detox to start buprenorphine, but you need to let yourself go into mild withdrawal before you take the first dose. After that you will not have any more withdrawal as long as you keep taking buprenorphine every day.

Like methadone, buprenorphine can be taken once a day, but you can take the medication at home. You can also get buprenorphine at a methadone clinic, but then you will need to come more often. Staff at the clinic will watch to make sure you take your dose. When you start taking buprenorphine and stop using illicit opioids, you may feel some craving and mild withdrawal for about a week or two. As with methadone, the different feelings can take some getting used to at the start of treatment.

Buprenorphine is safer and has fewer side effects than methadone. Some people still have cravings on buprenorphine. Higher doses may help reduce cravings. Buprenorphine may be a good first choice to try as a treatment. If you find a doctor who is able to prescribe it, you can start taking it almost immediately—you do not have to wait to get accepted into a methadone program or to go through a full detox.

Starting Methadone or Buprenorphine

Many people are concerned about having to stop heroin or pain-killer use before taking methadone or buprenorphine. It is true that it is not a good idea to take the medication when you are high on heroin. If you have used heroin recently and you take methadone, you may feel very sedated. If you take buprenorphine, you can go into withdrawal. It is best to be in a mild withdrawal when you take the first dose of either medication.

To safely start methadone, you only need to be abstinent over-night, for eight to twelve hours, or until you start feeling uncomfortable.

To safely start buprenorphine, you need to be abstinent for at least twelve to sixteen hours—usually the evening and night before you plan to start the medication. To start buprenorphine safely, it is not enough to feel anxious. You need to wait until you start feeling muscle aches, abdominal cramps, feel hot or cold, and start yawning. That way, the first dose of buprenorphine will make you feel better rather than worse.

When in doubt, wait. If you were using fentanyl or street methadone, you may actually need to wait about twenty-four hours before starting medication. Your withdrawal should still be mild, but you can take over-the-counter medications or ask the doctor to prescribe some.

Buprenorphine may help you more if you go to see a therapist trained to work with people taking buprenorphine.

Naltrexone

The medication naltrexone is not an opioid. It is an opioid blocker. Before you start it, you need to be fully detoxed. Unlike methadone and buprenorphine, naltrexone does not keep you physically dependent on opioids.

Naltrexone has no noticeable effect on your mood, but the medication decreases cravings. Naltrexone helps to prevent relapse. The medication blocks all of the opioid receptors in your brain so that you cannot get high from opioids. In other words, if you take heroin or painkillers, naltrexone will stop them from having any effect at all. You can take one naltrexone tablet every day, two or three tablets every two or three days, or one injection every four weeks. The injection works best for most people.

It may take a few weeks to get used to naltrexone if you start it right after your detox. You might continue to go through a mild withdrawal and have problems sleeping. If you start it after several weeks of abstinence, you will not have to get used to naltrexone.

Naltrexone has its pros and cons.

Pros:
- You will be protected against relapse.
- You will avoid overdose and death.
- You will stop obsessing about finding drugs.
- It is safe, with no risk of overdose.
- If you stop using it, you will not experience withdrawal.
- It is not a controlled substance; the doctor does not need a special license to prescribe it.
- Using it to prevent relapse is generally less controversial than using methadone or buprenorphine, both of which are opioids.

Cons:
- You need to be detoxed fully before you can start naltrexone.
- Usual doses of opioid painkillers will not work.

- You can overdose if you stop taking naltrexone and start using opioids again.
- It may take a few weeks to get used to naltrexone. You might continue to go through a mild withdrawal and have problems sleeping initially.

Naltrexone treatment cannot start until seven to ten days after you have taken your last opioid—you must go through a complete detox first. Taking naltrexone before opioids are completely out of your system causes instant and severe withdrawal. Never start naltrexone treatment without seeking medical advice.

Going through a complete detox is a hurdle for some people. If you can go to a detox center or residential treatment for the detox only, you are more likely to be successful starting naltrexone. But many people detox at home successfully, especially if they have a plan.

If you attempt to use while on naltrexone with the intention of "overriding the blockade," you may not feel anything at first, but very large doses of heroin may overpower the blockade, and you may overdose and die. If you stop taking naltrexone and relapse, you will be at a very high risk of overdosing. Because your body has been detoxed, it will be very sensitive to the effects of opioids on breathing. Even a small dose of a painkiller might be enough to cause breathing to stop. If you stop taking naltrexone and use heroin, you can die from an overdose. That is why it is so important to stay on naltrexone for as long as possible. It has few side effects and is very safe, even when used for a long time.

Detoxification Before Starting Naltrexone

If you plan to start naltrexone, you must first go through a full detoxification before you can take the medication. If you have detoxed before, look back on past detoxes to see what worked and what didn't work. Each time you detox, the experience is different, but some of the key symptoms that were present before may return. Be prepared for them.

Most people fear detox and therefore the natural tendency is to postpone it. The same happens with a diet or exercise routine. There is never a best time to start it. Although you will need to make some preparations—for example, getting time off work or the help of a supportive person—it makes no sense to postpone it for a long time. When using, things only get worse, so there is an urgency to stop using and get on with your plan.

Detox Don'ts

These two rules of detox are very important:

- *Don't* attempt detox unless you have a scheduled appointment with a doctor to go on XR-naltrexone after your detox. The medication prevents you from relapsing. Without medication to support your abstinence from opioids, you may be doing more harm than good by detoxing.

- *Don't* start using opioids when you are almost done with detox. You can easily overdose because you will be very sensitive to them. The doses you were using a week earlier may now shut down your breathing.

Where to Detox

Detoxing from opioids can be very uncomfortable, but it is usually not dangerous. Many people can safely detox at home on their own with over-the-counter medications. A medical detox is more comfortable because you will be given prescription medications to help with withdrawal symptoms. Let's look more closely at the options.

Inpatient detox

Detoxing in the hospital under medical supervision can be useful. The doctor will give you effective medications to help ease withdrawal symptoms. You can get medical attention if you need it. You also will not be able to stop the detox by taking heroin or another opioid. Try to detox in a hospital if you are in any of the following situations:

- Detoxing from alcohol or sedative drugs (Xanax, Valium) and opioids
- Have a medical disorder, such as diabetes, asthma, or hypertension
- Have tried and failed detox at home
- Have a history of overdosing after detox

Outpatient detox

Medical detox is also available at some outpatient drug treatment centers. Staff will give you prescription medications to make detox more tolerable and safer. Staff will also monitor your health. But you do not have to spend all day and night at the center. Outpatient detox is easier with the support of a loved one to bring you to visits and help monitor your take-home medications. Outpatient detox is a good choice if you do *not* have the following:

- Access to inpatient detox
- Insurance, or your insurance does not cover detox
- A week to spend in a hospital (because of work or caregiving duties)

Staff may be able to slow down your detox if you find the symptoms are too difficult to tolerate. Finally, the medical team that is supervising your detox may be the same team that will supervise your treatment with naltrexone. This continuity of care is helpful.

Residential treatment

A residential program (rehab) is a very good choice if you are planning to start relapse prevention treatment with naltrexone. The first week of residential treatment is usually focused on managing opioid withdrawal. Most programs offer medications to relieve withdrawal. After that, you will have a chance to settle into a drug-free state for another week or two before you receive the first injection of naltrexone. Your caregivers will monitor you for another week after that. Because you cannot get your drug of choice while in rehab, it is the best place to start naltrexone, although it is expensive.

At home

Many people detox at home or at a loved one's home. When you detox without medical supervision, ask friends, family, or a partner to help you. Have them see the doctor with you and talk about what your plans are after detox. Do not involve your using friends. This will make it harder for you not to use.

At home, you will enjoy the comfort of your own bed, shower, and bathroom. You can sleep and eat when you want. But it can be hard to make changes at home, especially if you used at home. You can do things ahead of time to prepare for detoxing at home:

- Stay somewhere comfortable with supportive people around you.
- Tell people close to you what you are planning to do.
- Clean your house before you start, make sure to get rid of all alcohol, drugs, and drug paraphernalia.
- Take time off work or school—ask your doctor for a sick note or take vacation time.
- Stock up on medications used to relieve flu symptoms and make sure you know how to use them.
- Have plenty of fluids on hand: sports drinks and warm broth are the best.
- Stock the kitchen with easy-to-digest foods and snacks, such as crackers, Jell-O, and plain toast.
- Collect movies to watch, games to play, and other things to occupy your time.
- Treat yourself as you would if you had a bad flu (but you are getting prepared for it rather than surprised by it).

Withdrawal symptoms begin about six to eight hours after you take your last opioid. Symptoms peak on days three and four, may go up or down, and usually disappear before the week is over. If you take medication, your symptoms may be milder but will last about the same length of time.

It is good to have a detox plan. For example, you will stay at home for a week and take medications every day to help with withdrawal. When you are finished detoxing, you will go to the doctor to get a naltrexone injection. Make sure the doctor is expecting you and has the injection ready.

But you also need a contingency plan. If things don't go well—if you are confused and disoriented, dizzy and prone to falling, depressed or suicidal—you need to go to the emergency room. You can also change your mind. You can abandon the plan of completing the detox and start treatment with methadone or buprenorphine. Before you detox, explore where you will go for these medications.

If you do not finish your detox and take painkillers or heroin, you can easily overdose. Start with very small doses.

Detox produces profound changes in your body. You will be purging the drugs from your body, and this will take a toll on you. Feeling at least a little sick is unavoidable. Some people say that if you feel lousy, that means that detox is working and that your body is going through needed changes. Detox is easier to deal with if you accept it rather than avoiding it or fighting it. Feeling sick is part of your healing—and it is temporary.

CHAPTER 12

The First Days and Weeks After You Stop Using

I want you to be prepared for what will happen to you when you stop taking heroin or painkillers. Even if you start taking medication that contains opioids and do not go through detox, you will experience changes. You will feel a difference in your body, your thoughts, your feelings, and your relationships. At first, these changes may feel strange or uncomfortable. Eventually, you will begin to feel much better.

The changes you go through will be milder and more gradual if you start with methadone or buprenorphine. If you decide to take naltrexone, the changes may be more intense initially. You will also need to go through some of these changes if you decide to transition from methadone onto buprenorphine or from buprenorphine onto naltrexone.

Some people do not want to make too many changes at once. They may find naltrexone very attractive but need time to prepare for detox first. If you feel this way, you can start with buprenorphine first and then after a few weeks transition onto naltrexone. This more gradual transition may be easier to cope with.

If you know what to expect in treatment, you can more easily deal with the changes. Any withdrawal symptoms or change you experience will be less severe if you are prepared for them. Not knowing what to expect makes some people anxious. Being anxious can make withdrawal symptoms feel worse. If you talk through your feelings about withdrawal and going on medication, you are more likely to get off and remain abstinent from opioids.

Talk about the options with a supportive person or your doctor. They can help you choose the right option for you at this time.

What Happens to Your Body

Using opioids regularly changed some of your bodily functions. You may have gotten used to being constipated, having little energy, needing a lot of sleep, and not being able to function sexually. Now, your body must reset and adjust to functioning without your drug of choice. When your body is resetting itself, you experience withdrawal symptoms.

Experiencing withdrawal is like having a really bad case of the flu. To feel better, you can use over-the-counter medications used to treat the flu, such as those that help with headaches and muscle aches, upset stomach, nausea, vomiting, diarrhea, and insomnia.

Here are some common withdrawal symptoms. You may already know them. But detoxifying as part of treatment is different than getting sick when you do not have enough drugs at home. You might have different symptoms or fewer symptoms. Usually, withdrawal is less severe. Very often, my patients are surprised at how they feel, as they were prepared for much worse. It is just good to be prepared for what might happen.

- Anxiety
- Irritability
- Cold shakes and sweats
- Restlessness

- Muscle aches
- Diarrhea
- Yawning
- Poor sleep
- Nausea
- Vomiting
- Watery eyes/runny nose

What Happens to Your Thoughts and Feelings

Opioid use numbs all feelings, good and bad. When you are using, all your pain, stress, and worries disappear. If disturbing feelings come back, you can quickly send them away with another dose of heroin. Once you stop the constant and excessive flow of opioids to your brain, suddenly all your emotions come to the surface. In recovery, all your emotions come back to life. You will feel painful emotions as well as pleasurable emotions—sadness and joy, fear and laughter. These will be your real emotions.

Because you are no longer turning to drugs to deal with emotions, you need to slowly experience the world of intense emotions and gradually learn how to rein them in. You can take advantage of these emotions. They are your signals to the world around you.

At first, you might feel as if you are on a long, fast roller-coaster ride that has all the biggest highs and lows at the beginning. Things usually settle down as you get used to coping with the emotions and feelings. However, you will likely have second thoughts and wish to go back to the familiar, comforting feeling that comes with using opioids. Riding the wave of emotions is one of the many challenges of recovery. Over time, most people like experiencing this new world of feelings.

These fresh experiences may be particularly strong if you go through a complete detoxification and start taking naltrexone. There will be highs, but also lows, and at times depression may set in for longer than moments or days. You may experience fewer emotional ups and downs with methadone or buprenorphine, but how much you will feel is hard to predict.

People react differently to coming off opioids, so be prepared to experience a range of new feelings that will be mostly bad, though some may be good. You may feel unhappy or depressed, anxious, or irritable. You may have rushes of emotion, laugh hysterically, or go through crying spells. You may feel bored or tired.

Your thoughts will likely change as well. You might have a lot of uncomfortable thoughts. You might keep thinking or obsessing about drugs or other things. You may feel confused or not as sharp as you used to be. You also might remember bad things that happened while you were using or before you started using.

Having so many feelings and thoughts can make you want to use again. It might help to tell yourself that things are worse now because you have just made a huge change. Remind yourself that there may be things you want to sort out. When you give it some time, these thoughts and feelings start to settle down.

Be mindful of your thoughts. Just thinking about heroin can create physical withdrawal symptoms. The opposite is also true: If you think about how good life can be in recovery, withdrawal symptoms may lessen.

What Happens to Your Relationships

When you were using, the people around you saw you as being very different from the person they once knew. They may have distanced themselves from you, stopped trusting you, and even given up on you. In recovery, the people around you have to adjust to the new you. This can take time. Do not be surprised if some people have a hard time trusting you at first or are angry.

At the same time, you will likely lose your using friends. They will feel uncomfortable being around someone who is not using. If you hang out with them while they are using, you will feel tempted to use.

The beginning of treatment is a good time to build a network of friends who are not using. For example, you may want to check out local self-help groups. Narcotics Anonymous (NA) is an organization run by people who used narcotics and now want to help others stop. Alcoholics Anonymous (AA) groups, which use the same Twelve Step model, are much easier to find and can also be helpful. You will find a lot of support in those meetings, a new group of people to spend time with, and trusted friends. Connections you develop by going to the meetings can be very strong and lasting. Many members have been sober for a long time, so they know how difficult recovery can be.

Support groups do not suit everyone. You may not like the idea of sharing your problems with strangers. You may not like how the groups are run. Most groups require that you be free of all mood-altering drugs, including alcohol and cannabis, and some groups may not be accepting of medications, such as methadone or buprenorphine, that help you stay abstinent. SMART Recovery groups may be more accepting of medication-based paths to recovery than traditional groups based on the Twelve Step model.

Staying on, Changing, or Stopping Medication

Understand and consider all your options before you make a decision about which medication to use or how to detox. Discuss the choice with your family and with a doctor or a therapist who understands the options. You might also want to reach out to people like yourself who are using medication to treat opioid addiction.

Staying on medication

Once you choose a medication, it is important to take it as prescribed. Sometimes people get their family members or partners to give them the tablets in the morning. You can ask a relative or a sober friend to go with you for your monthly injection or daily methadone dosage, or take your tablet with your doctor or therapist. These are ways of increasing your resolve to stay on the path of recovery. Most people are better about taking their medication on time when supervised. In the end, however, there is no substitute for taking responsibility for yourself.

Changing dosage or medication

If you do not care for the medication you start taking in treatment, talk to your doctor. If you still have cravings, do not feel well, or have side effects that are hard to manage, you can talk about trying a different dosage of the medication. Or you can ask to try a different medication.

Stopping medication

If you start feeling confident that you can stop taking your medication and remain abstinent, continue to take your medication. Always talk to your doctor before stopping a medication—and always have a plan for what to do next. Many people start to feel good, quit taking their medicine, and relapse. If you are feeling good and doing well, that means the medication is working. It is a sign that you should stay on it. Once you stop the medication, your cravings and drug obsessions may return.

You may feel pressure from family members or friends from self-help groups to stop taking your medication. They might think that if your medicine is an opioid, you are not really in recovery. They might tell you that you are now addicted to pills because you have to take them every day.

Most people do not understand how opioid addiction works. And they do not understand how deadly relapse to today's strong opioids can be. Do not let these people confuse you. If your medication is working well and you are doing better, you should stay on the medication. If you start getting pressure to stop medication from family members, ask them to come to the doctor with you. The doctor can explain why the medication is necessary.

Addiction is a chronic, lifelong disorder. There is no shame in taking medication to treat a chronic illness. If you would accept having to take insulin injections every day for diabetes or medication to keep HIV from becoming AIDS, you can feel grateful about taking medication for addiction.

How to Stay Sober

Overdose and your new tolerance level

Accidental overdose following detox in people who do not start medication is one of the most common causes of death for people with opioid addiction.

If you underwent a complete detox, your tolerance to opioids is back at zero. Quantities of opioids that would have "done nothing" to you before detoxification could now kill you. Even 30 mg of oxycodone or two bags of heroin can be fatal once you have lost your tolerance to opioids. Keep naloxone (Narcan) nearby even after treatment. Taking medication protects you from overdosing on painkillers or heroin, but you can still overdose on other drugs. Mixing alcohol with sedatives, such as Xanax, makes even small amounts of opioids deadly. Taking counterfeit pills, such as those that may contain fentanyl, can also be deadly, even during buprenorphine, methadone, or naltrexone treatment. Fentanyl can sometimes bust through the medication.

Cravings and triggers

The desire to use opioids can take you by surprise. It may happen even if you are taking medication, but much more so if you are not. If you want to overcome cravings, be prepared. Keep a list of people to call and things you can do to stay active during a craving.

In therapy, you learn strategies for dealing with strong craving. You can tell others about it or distract your mind by turning your attention to an activity. You can leave the house or go to the gym for an intensive workout. Try recalling all the negative consequences of using and what could happen if you decide to use this time. It is useful to write those down, on your phone or on an index card you keep in your wallet. When craving comes, you can look at this list and imagine each of those things happening to you. Cravings do not last forever.

You will naturally link all sorts of people, places, and things with using. These people, places, and things are known as triggers. Every person addicted to drugs has their own unique list of triggers. If you want to protect yourself against relapse, it is essential that you spend time creating a list of your triggers. Write them down and keep your list on you. As time goes on, you will probably discover more triggers. Knowing what they are is the first step to overcoming them. The second step is avoiding them.

Common triggers include certain objects, such as money in your pocket; certain places or bars; and being around using friends and drug paraphernalia or prescription bottles. Feelings can also be powerful triggers. Feeling stressed or overwhelmed, angry after an argument, or bored or disappointed can also make you think about using. Even memories and dreams can trigger a desire to use.

Each time you recognize and cope with a triggered craving, the trigger gets a little easier to deal with the next time. Do not let yourself get complacent, though. And do not intentionally expose yourself to high-risk situations or people. You will change from day to day. A situation you coped with easily one day may cause a stronger craving the next time. Triggers will lose their strength over time. Allow this to happen naturally.

Lapse

A lapse is a temporary return to using, usually once or a few times. If you use and then decide you want to stop, you probably won't suffer physical withdrawal symptoms because of the opioid use. If you lapse while taking medication, you will probably not have withdrawal symptoms. You may suffer anxiety, worry, or physical symptoms caused by the stress of remembering what withdrawals are like.

Do not be afraid to ask for help. You are not letting people down if you do. A lapse is not a disaster or proof you can't stay in recovery. A lapse is an opportunity to work through what happened. It shows you what you need to do differently.

Most lapses will turn into relapses unless you deal with them at once. Your best defense is to talk to your doctor and take your medication, which will block the effects of the drugs, stopping the lapse from becoming a relapse.

Relapse

If you use for longer than two weeks, on most days, and you cannot stop on your own, you have relapsed. When you relapse, you may feel as if you are back at square one. But if you have learned from the experience, you will be wiser. You will know what you need to do differently so that you can stay in recovery.

Ask for help. Many people who have been off opioids for years will tell you that they relapsed several times. If you follow your treatment recommendations, you minimize the risk of relapse. But you cannot fully protect yourself against it. Do not blame yourself. If you relapse, talk to your doctor about next steps.

Establish a New Mind-set

The more problems you have, the stronger the urge to use becomes, and the more difficult it is to resist. It is easier to stay off opioids if you are clear with yourself that, no matter what happens, you will not use. Opioids are no longer an option. That way, instead of asking yourself whether things are bad enough to justify using, you will be asking yourself how you are going to cope.

CHAPTER 13

The Next Months and Years Once You Are Drug-Free

Addiction is a lifelong disorder. Although there is no cure for opioid use disorder (OUD), you can learn to live with it. Millions of people who have chronic disorders live full lives by learning to manage them.

The first stage of treatment requires getting used to your medication. You are getting stable. At some point, you realize that you no longer have opioid cravings or think obsessively about using. You are abstinent and no longer have problems related to opioid use, such as withdrawals or cravings.

Once you achieve initial success in treatment, you will want to maintain it by taking your medication and abstaining from drugs and alcohol. Once you can manage your disorder, and can live a full life in spite of it, you are in what we call recovery. Usually, recovery is defined as a place you get to after you complete treatment. I prefer to think of recovery as a next stage of treatment because, with chronic disorders, there is no end to treatment. You will need to check in with a therapist or doctor to get medication and monitor how you are doing.

In this next phase, your focus shifts from trying to stay off drugs to being productive and making life enjoyable and even exciting. Now you can focus on improving your health and quality of life. You can also do things to reduce the risk of relapse to opioid use.

In this chapter, you will learn what to expect in recovery, as well as some tools to help you stay in recovery. Recovery from addiction is often referred to as a journey that can take you to interesting places. I like to talk about recovery as taking a journey on a train.

The Four Wheels of the Recovery Train

The recovery train you are on has four wheels. Each wheel does its job to support the train and keep it on track. With four good wheels, the train is powerful and fast. It is able to go through various obstacles along the way. If one of the wheels falls off, the train is shaky and less stable. If a second wheel falls off, it doesn't matter how strong or durable the other two wheels are. The train can still move but not for long. With only one wheel, the trip will be very short before it crashes. With only one or even two wheels the train has little chance of making it to its destination. The journey is over until the wheels can be repaired. The four wheels of the recovery train are as follows:

1. Engage in treatment.
2. Take maintenance medication.
3. Maintain abstinence.
4. Build a satisfying life.

A successful and enduring recovery requires that you keep all of the wheels in working order. You must check and maintain them regularly to ensure you will have a safe and enjoyable ride for years to come.

Wheel 1: Engage in treatment

Most people accept that they need to go to a medical doctor for an annual exam, whether they like it or not. When people are sick or injured, they need to go for additional visits, sometimes quite often, until the problem is resolved. If they keep all their appointments, their illness resolves itself as quickly as possible. Once they feel better, they check in with the doctor once in a while, but at least once a year. They want to make sure they maintain their health and catch any problems early so the doctor can intervene before it is too late.

You can look at treatment sessions the same way. If you accept that you must go to each treatment session, whether you feel sick or well, it is easier. After the first phase of addiction treatment is over, you will want to go regularly for recovery checkups, with a therapist and a doctor. Checkups can stop problems from becoming reasons to use. You can talk through stressful life events with a therapist, which can help you to see things differently. You can learn how to deal with them. Having someone help you monitor your health and progress can be comforting. It's also good to keep an open mind. If your therapist or doctor recommends a different level of care, think about how it might help you.

You can also attend self-help groups, such as Narcotics Anonymous (NA) or Alcoholics Anonymous (AA). Go to a meeting at least four times before you decide how you feel about it. Being around other people in recovery helps many people stay sober. Being a regular and active participant in those groups can be extremely helpful.

The key to success is to stay engaged and do it even if you are in good health and may think you do not need it anymore. Make sure your treatment team knows how to find you and that you keep them informed. If you decide to move, let them know so they can help you find another team near your new home.

Wheel 2: Take maintenance medication

Medication is another important wheel. Without medication, your recovery train is on shaky ground. It can still go but much slower and less safely. Medication helped you a lot at the beginning of the journey. Who knows where you would be without it. If your medication helped you in the past, why give it up? Why question it or try going without it?

If you experience side effects or have other problems with your medication, talk to your doctor. Do not wait too long. Sometimes, all you need is a simple change. The doctor might adjust the dose or offer a different form of the same medication.

If you keep forgetting to take your medication or find it a nuisance, your doctor might recommend a long-acting injection or an implant. If you feel like the medication is not working as well as it used to—maybe you have a dream about using or start noticing cravings—tell your doctor. The doctor might put you on a different medication. Some people have to try all three medications before they find the one that works best for them. The doctor will help you manage any problems, but you need to communicate them.

If a loved one or a close friend is encouraging you to stop taking your medication, bring them to the doctor with you. The doctor can explain why medication is important.

If you feel "normal" but you do not want to take your medication because of side effects or cost, talk to your doctor about changing to another medication. You can also discuss the possibility of tapering off. The doctor will help you decide whether this is a good idea and whether you are ready. Keep taking your medication until you've talked to the doctor about tapering. People who stay on medication for as long as possible do better than people who stop taking it.

Wheel 3: Maintain sobriety

Sobriety is a big part of recovery. Sobriety means being free of opioids and other intoxicating substances. Many professionals and people with a history of addiction believe that people who take medications, such as methadone or buprenorphine, are not sober. These views have started to change, especially with the dramatic rise in opioid overdose deaths in the past few years.

More and more people accept the view that a person taking medication to stay abstinent from opioids is sober as long as they are abstinent from all other drugs and alcohol and do not have any symptoms of any substance use disorder.

Tobacco, one of the most addictive and harmful substances, is given special treatment for the time being. For now, people who are only addicted to tobacco are still considered to be in recovery.

Some people start to think that after a long abstinence they are due for a "treat" or that using opioids once in a while will not hurt. This "addictive thinking" is detrimental to recovery. The drug experience is powerful. If you take opioids again, you are likely to backslide into your old patterns of use, because your brain is still the same as the brain that was operating when you were addicted. The longer the gap since you last used, the slower the slide. But if you use and think it will be "just this once," and that you will be able to stop before it gets bad, the chances of relapse are high. People can quickly resume using regularly even after five or more years in recovery.

If you decide to try opioids again while on your medication, you will be protected from relapse. If you stop taking your medication to use opioids, you are no longer protected against relapse. In addition, you will be at high risk of overdose.

Abstinence also means staying away from drugs that are not your "drug of choice." Alcohol or other drugs can weaken your commitment to recovery and make it harder for you to resist opioids. Some prescription medications may also be problematic for people who want to maintain sobriety. Always mention your OUD to the prescribing doctor and discuss the benefits and risks of taking these medications.

Wheel 4: Build a satisfying life

Recovery is about making your life better. In recovery, you have time to do new things. Fill this time with people, work, and activities that are meaningful to you. Join groups that interest you, whether political, humanitarian, or spiritual.

Seek out supportive family and friends. Tell them you are working on your recovery and ask if they can help you stay on track.

Look for a job that you find rewarding. Job centers can help you discover what types of things you like to do. You might enjoy work that requires a lot of physical activity, for instance, or a job that uses organizing skills.

Health is always a priority. Exercise and stay active doing things you enjoy. The more you like it, the more you will do it. Find people to exercise with. Working out or staying active with others is fun and keeps you accountable.

Take care of your body by eating healthy foods. Stay away from junk or fast foods. The kind of food you eat affects how you feel physically and even mentally. The better you feel, the more you will want to stay in recovery.

If necessary, improve the quality of your living situation. Look for a place to live that is safe and stable and in a neighborhood free of violence and drugs. Look for roommates who do not use or are in recovery.

It may feel strange at first. Some people feel as if they are halfway between one way of life and another. You will eventually gain more confidence in your new life. People who do not have addiction do the same kinds of things to make their lives better. Everyone struggles sometimes. It is up to each person to build a satisfying life.

If you start to think that one part of your recovery no longer matters, remember the train analogy. Recovery is better and easier when you maintain all four wheels so you can confidently continue on your journey.

Going through a crisis such as addiction is an opportunity for growth. In recovery, you come out stronger, more mature, and more "human." This is a time for you to look more closely at yourself and do things that align with your values. When you are true to yourself, the world opens up to you in ways you never expected.

EPILOGUE: OVERDOSES AS MISSED OPPORTUNITIES

Many communities have established programs to save individuals with naloxone postoverdose. This saves lives initially but does little to prevent future overdoses, which will likely happen in most people rescued with naloxone. These people are at highest risk of overdosing again, and they are rarely able to connect with and start adequate treatment. They get up, thank their rescuer, and walk away to resume use because no one has addressed the disorder. This is similar to treating a broken arm in an alcoholic who fell on the ice while drunk. Casting the arm does nothing to prevent it from happening again because the root of the problem is not being addressed. Why not stop overdoses before they occur? About one in twenty opioid overdoses on any given day is fatal, and the average person who overdoses goes on to have ten to twenty overdose events. These near deaths serve as a dozen or more missed opportunities for shepherding someone into treatment with methadone, buprenorphine, or injectable naltrexone, the three FDA-approved medications proven effective in reducing overdoses. When opioid overdose victims are offered treatment with buprenorphine in the emergency room and they accept it, they initially do better than people only given a phone number to call.

Naloxone is necessary, but I am afraid that on its own it is merely a Band-Aid. Focusing efforts on it may distract policy makers from seeking needed solutions. Naloxone works best as part of a comprehensive treatment system, where overdoses can be reversed but, more importantly, prevented. If only naloxone advocates could mobilize their enthusiasm and resources to expand their mission to increase information and access to maintenance treatments with methadone, buprenorphine, or naltrexone—a more complex but ultimately lifesaving task.

With the rapid expansion of fentanyl-like drugs and other powerful opioids, the call for evidence-based treatment is now more urgent than ever. In just three short years, between 2013 and 2016, US deaths from fentanyl rose by 540 percent. When people overdose on fentanyl, naloxone only makes a tiny impact. Heroin leaves a longer timeframe, depending on how much is consumed, during which the antidote can be administered successfully. With fentanyl, breathing stops in a matter of minutes, and rescuers have little time to deliver the antidote. The only hope in protecting individuals from death by fentanyl is to have easy access to OUD medications. The unique situation we find ourselves in calls for a new paradigm—long-term medical treatment as an overdose-reduction strategy.

Treating Waves Three and Four of the Epidemic

The opioid epidemic is currently in its third wave: It started with the explosion of prescription painkiller use between 2000 and 2010. It moved on to heroin. Since 2013, we have seen a dramatic rise in fentanyl use. Current treatment approaches using medications were developed and designed for the first and second phases of the epidemic. We do not know whether these treatments will be adequate to help individuals addicted to fentanyl or whether we can prevent fentanyl overdose deaths. Fentanyl-like substances appear to be different enough from heroin or painkillers that patients using them regularly may need a different treatment approach. Currently, there are no studies to help guide treatment, yet fentanyl is particularly deadly, and additional research is urgently needed if this trend continues.

A fourth wave of the epidemic may be on the rise, one that is already being seen in other countries and in some parts of the United States. An increasing number of people are using opioids in combination with stimulants and establishing a mixed opioid/stimulant addiction. In increasing numbers, opioid users are adding cocaine and methamphetamine to the mix. Treating such individuals will require yet a different strategy. Methadone, buprenorphine, and naltrexone work well for OUD, but other drugs are not fazed by the medications. Less is known about medications that can help reduce cravings for and use of stimulants.

I would not be surprised if within another thirty years we have a test to tell who is at high risk of developing addiction. We will have vaccines to protect people at the highest risk and to prevent relapse in people who achieve initial abstinence. We will have many more medications to safely treat addictions to all substances, including long-acting medicines, an injection that only has to be taken once or twice per year, or perhaps an implant lasting a lifetime. We will have tests to tell which medication to use for any given patient. We will use physical treatments—magnetic, electric, or light stimulation—to diminish functioning in very select areas of the brain to decrease or eliminate craving and improve decision-making in afflicted individuals.

But for now, the urgency to treat existing OUD patients with the effective medication we have on hand is at an all-time high. If we catch opioid users before they turn to fentanyl-like opioids or stimulants, we can profoundly reduce the impact of the next waves—which we are less prepared to tackle than we are opioids as a single addiction. When the fourth wave crests, the nation will be drowning in an even bigger sea of overdoses.

Methadone

Medication names: Methadose, Diskets, Dolophine

Administration: Oral liquid, tablet, tablet for suspension

How it works: Methadone fully activates opioid receptors in the brain.

What it does: Patients taking methadone have less craving and they use less heroin or prescription opioids, stay in treatment longer, and have fewer medical complications, lower risk of death, and improved social and work functioning.

Where to get it: Only available in licensed opioid treatment programs (OTPs). Methadone is a controlled substance (schedule II). It can only be used legally by a person enrolled in an OTP. Methadone tablets available by prescription from the pharmacy cannot be used for the treatment of opioid withdrawal and OUD maintenance.

Detoxification: Detoxification is not required before starting methadone. Methadone acts as an opioid and patients treated with it will remain physically dependent. If taken daily, methadone prevents withdrawal, but if abruptly stopped, opioid withdrawal will begin within 36–48 hours.

Wait time: No wait time or withdrawal symptoms required before first dose is given, but the patient cannot be intoxicated or sedated.

Dosing: Lower doses (20–40 mg/day) are sufficient to eliminate physical withdrawal; 50–60 mg doses eliminate subjective withdrawal and craving; higher doses (60–120 mg) are needed to block the effects of heroin and decrease the risk of opioid use.

Lag time to full effect: Methadone has to be started with a low dose and increased slowly; it may take 2 or more weeks before a fully therapeutic dose is reached.

Possible side effects: Sedation during treatment initiation, dizziness, constipation, nausea/vomiting, excessive sweating, low blood pressure

Serious adverse effects: Heart arrhythmia or deep somnolence with slowing of breathing, both of which may result in death

Contraindications: Acute asthma, severe breathing problems, obstruction of bowels

Blockade: High doses of methadone (above 100 mg) are more effective in blocking illicit opioids but may not be sufficient to block very high doses of heroin or fentanyl.

Overdose risk: If the daily dose is increased too fast at the beginning of treatment; if a high dose of methadone is taken in combination with high doses of other sedatives such as benzodiazepines, sleep medicines (especially if injected), or alcohol; after methadone is abruptly stopped and heroin use is resumed, especially after several days of no opioids.

Potential for abuse: Methadone can be abused if taken in higher doses, in combination with sedatives, or injected.

Limitations: Only available at specialty clinics with restrictive regulations; medications must be taken daily at the clinic during early stages of treatment.

Buprenorphine

Buprenorphine mono products

Tablet: Sublingual: various generic products

Injection: Subcutaneous: Subcolade monthly injection under the skin of the abdomen

Implant: Subcutaneous: Probuphine for surgical implantation under the skin on the upper arm, to be removed and replaced every 6 months

Buprenorphine combination products (buprenorphine with naloxone)

Film: Sublingual: Suboxone, to be placed under the tongue

Film: Buccal: Bunavail, to be attached inside the mouth on the cheek

Tablet: Sublingual: Zubsolv, and various generic tablets

Other preparations with buprenorphine (film or skin patch) cannot be used for treatment of OUD.

How it works: Buprenorphine partially activates opioid receptors in the brain; works similarly to methadone.

What it does: Patients taking buprenorphine have less craving and use less heroin or prescription opioids, stay in treatment longer, have reduced risk of overdose, lower use of other drugs, overall lower addiction severity, and improved functioning.

Where to get it: Available in opioid treatment programs or from a medical provider (MD or DO physician, physician assistant, or a nurse practitioner) authorized by the DEA to use buprenorphine products approved for OUD. Buprenorphine is a controlled substance (schedule III). It can only be used by a person with a prescription; giving it to another person is illegal.

Detoxification: Detoxification is not required before starting buprenorphine. Buprenorphine acts as an opioid, and patients treated with it will remain physically dependent. If taken daily, buprenorphine prevents withdrawal. If abruptly stopped, opioid withdrawal will begin 36–48 hours later; the severity of withdrawal will be mild.

Wait time: The patient has to be in the early stages of opioid withdrawal before taking the first dose of buprenorphine: 12 hours for heroin, 24 hours for long-acting painkillers or fentanyl, and 48 hours or longer in the case of methadone.

Dosing: Lower doses (2–8 mg/day) are sufficient to eliminate physical and subjective withdrawal; doses of 12–24 mg eliminate craving, block the effects of heroin, and decrease risk of opioid use.

Lag time to full effect: The first dose is usually low (2 mg) to make sure it can be tolerated; over the first one to three days, the dosage can be increased rapidly if needed to control symptoms, to 16–24 mg/day.

Possible side effects: Sedation during treatment initiation, dizziness, headache, constipation, abdominal pain, nausea, excessive sweating, and low blood pressure. Site where injection is given or implant is placed may be tender or painful, with possibility of itching, redness, or swelling.

Serious adverse effects: Low blood pressure (rare); injecting buprenorphine, especially in combination with other sedatives, may cause slowing of breathing, overdose, and death.

Contraindications: Acute asthma, severe breathing problems, obstruction of bowels

Blockade: Higher doses of buprenorphine (24–32 mg) are more effective in blocking illicit opioids but may not be sufficient to block very high doses of heroin or fentanyl.

Overdose risk: If buprenorphine is taken in combination with high doses of other sedatives such as benzodiazepines, sleep medicines, or alcohol, especially if buprenorphine is injected; after buprenorphine is abruptly stopped and heroin use is resumed, especially after several days of no opioids.

Potential for abuse: Buprenorphine can be abused through injection.

Limitations: Medical provider needs to be authorized to prescribe buprenorphine.

APPENDIX C:
QUICK GUIDE TO NALTREXONE

Naltrexone

Medication types

Tablet: By mouth: various generic products, 50 mg

Injection: (intramuscular; Vivitrol—one injection every 4 weeks deep into the buttock muscle)

Implant: (subcutaneous; various types of implants made by a pharmacist; can be implanted surgically). The FDA has not yet reviewed or approved the use of implants in the United States.

How it works: Naltrexone blocks opioid receptors in the brain without activating them. Naltrexone works differently from methadone and buprenorphine.

What it does: Naltrexone can only be used after detoxification to prevent relapse. Patients taking naltrexone have less craving for opioids, are less likely to relapse, and stay in treatment longer.

Where to get it: Available from any medical provider who can prescribe medications; no special authorization is needed. It is not a controlled substance.

Detoxification: Detoxification is required before starting naltrexone. Naltrexone acts as an opioid blocker and will precipitate withdrawal in patients who are still physically dependent. Patients treated with naltrexone are not physically dependent. If naltrexone is stopped, there is no withdrawal nor any discomfort.

Wait time: The patient has to be fully detoxified, which means that all withdrawal symptoms have to be resolved. This takes on average 7 days after the last dose of an opioid like heroin, but it may take 10–14 days after the last dose of methadone, buprenorphine, or fentanyl. In patients who receive methadone for detoxification, there may be a delay of 2–3 weeks from the last dose of heroin before naltrexone can be safely given.

Dosing: Naltrexone tablet (50 mg) can be given daily or 2–3 times per week in 100 or 150 mg doses (average dose per day of 50 mg). Adherence to oral naltrexone is very poor unless it is directly observed. Extended-release naltrexone is given as an injection every 4 weeks or once monthly. There is usually no need for a dose increase, though higher-than-recommended doses can be used if needed. There should be no delay between doses of XR-naltrexone; if the next dose is delayed or the patient is unable to come to the office, they should receive naltrexone tablets until the day of injection.

Lag time to full effect: Immediate effect, no need for a dose increase; with naltrexone tablets the maximum blocking effect occurs in 1–2 hours and the naltrexone injection reaches its maximum effect on day 2, with blocking effects already present 2 hours after the injection.

Possible side effects: If there is too short of a delay from the last dose of opioids, patients may experience withdrawal-like symptoms including insomnia, tiredness, agitation, anxiety, diarrhea, nausea, and loss of appetite. Headache may also occur. Mild withdrawal-like symptoms may occur during the first month after the first naltrexone injection. Patients may also develop anxiety or depression.

Serious adverse effects: If naltrexone is given to a person who is physically dependent on opioids, severe withdrawal may be precipitated, including agitation, severe anxiety, insomnia, and even disorientation and hallucinations. Precipitated withdrawal may last 1–2 days. Injection-site reaction may also occur, most commonly tenderness and itching; rarely, the injection site may become very painful with redness and swelling that may require surgical intervention. Injecting naltrexone very deep into the muscle reduces the risk of site reaction. Patients may develop an allergic reaction to the injection or develop severe pneumonia.

Contraindications: Naltrexone should not be used in patients who require treatment of pain with opioids.

Blockade: Standard doses of oral or injection naltrexone are usually sufficient to prevent craving or to block average doses of heroin or painkillers, but it may not be sufficient to block very high doses of heroin or fentanyl.

Overdose risk: Naltrexone by itself does not affect respiration. It will prevent overdose from opioids but will not prevent overdose from other sedatives or alcohol. Overdose can occur if the patient tries to override the blockade by using increasing doses of heroin to achieve euphoria. There is a risk of overdose after naltrexone is abruptly stopped and heroin use is resumed. The blockade wears off 2–3 days after the last dose of a naltrexone tablet and 5–6 weeks after the last dose of injection naltrexone. Patients should be informed about this risk often during treatment.

Potential for abuse: Naltrexone has no abuse potential.

Limitations: Medication is difficult to start in patients who actively use opioids.

ACKNOWLEDGMENTS

I would like to thank my coauthor, Karen Chernyaev, for her patience and support throughout the process of writing this book. Karen's experience as an editor of many books in the field of nonmedical addiction treatment was a great match with my intent to bring the scientific and medical knowledge to readers who may only be familiar with traditional treatment. Her ability to develop patients' stories and use them to illustrate complicated clinical issues made this book lively and hopefully much more interesting to read than it would be otherwise.

I am most grateful to my wife, Dr. Katarzyna Wlodarczyk Bisaga, for her unwavering emotional support through thirty years of my academic career, including the intense few months I devoted to the writing of this book. I am also grateful to my children for allowing me extra time away from our family life to work on the book.

There are so many colleagues to thank. Without them, I would not be where I am today. Most importantly, Dr. Herbert Kleber, the most generous, sincere, kind, and good-humored clinician and scientist I have ever worked with. He inspired me to devote my professional life to caring for people with substance use disorders—to take on working with this highly stigmatized population, see their humanity and unique needs, and be able to enjoy it. Special thanks to the late Dr. Marian Fischman, whose mentoring during my first few years at Columbia made an indelible impact on my thinking about the importance of scientific rigor in addiction research, which I hope to continue.

Two of my closest colleagues—those I've learned from most, and with whom I've shared my work on opioid addiction treatment— are Drs. Ned Nunes and Maria Sullivan. I am greatly indebted to both of them for their incisive minds and most generous spirits.

Many other colleagues in Columbia's Division on Substance Use Disorders have supported my research efforts; most importantly, Dr. Frances Levin, the division's director who supported my academic career, and the other colleagues with whom I spent more than twenty years conducting research at the Substance Use Research Service: Drs. Richard Foltin, Sandy Comer, Meg Haney, and Suzette Evans.

I would like to thank Drs. John Mariani and Ken Carpenter, with whom I spent countless hours, spread over more than fifteen years, thinking through many complex clinical problems and coming up with innovative research ideas. Finally, I would like to thank the whole STARS (Substance Treatment and Research Service) team, especially long-term research coordinator Kaitlyn Mishlen and the countless research assistants who have been patient enough to work with me over these years. The STARS team and spirit make it a great place to work and help make taking care of patients as a team so rewarding.

It has been a privilege for me to be involved in training so many stellar young addiction psychiatrists who have come to Columbia to learn the craft. Some of them became close collaborators, most recently Dr. Arthur Robin Williams, who has a bright and open mind and the excitement needed to push our field forward. He and I have worked closely on many topics that are discussed in this book, and I am thankful for his insight and support.

I would like to thank many professional colleagues outside of Columbia. Most importantly, Drs. Gilberto Gerra and Elizabeth Saenz, the two most wonderful and devoted physicians who made the Drug Prevention and Health Branch of the United Nations Office on Drugs and Crime (UNODC) a place that cares deeply about health and reaches the most needy populations in distant places across the globe. I am thankful for all the opportunities to work with the UNODC team in Vienna as well as in many other faraway places.

A few visionary clinicians I have met in the course of my professional life really stand out: most importantly, Drs. George O'Neil and Colin Brewer, who definitely taught me to think outside the box, and Percy Menzies, from whom I learned how to make helping addicted patients enjoyable.

I am also glad I met so many interesting professional colleagues during my work in the area of addiction treatment. My appreciation to Drs. Ed Salsitz and Sarah Church, who were my go-to methadone treatment experts; Dr. David Ockert, a naltrexone expert, and Drs. Charles O'Brien, Tom Kosten, and George Woody, with whom I had many fascinating discussions about medication development. And finally, Dr. Tom McLellan, who continues to inspire me and whose work and courage in changing the field of addiction treatment I hold in the highest esteem.

I am grateful for my colleagues and friends in Poland, where I started my work in addiction treatment almost thirty years ago, especially Drs. Piotr Popik, Marcin Wojnar, and Magdalena Borkowska. After all these years, we continue to collaborate and discuss new developments in our work. And talking to them helps me keep my work in a broader perspective.

I thank the National Institute on Drug Abuse for its ongoing financial support of my research for the past twenty years, which has allowed me to learn so much about addiction treatment and contributed to the writing of this book.

I extend a special thanks to Matthew Lore, president and publisher at The Experiment, who encouraged me to write this book and helped me to realize how important it would be. His tight deadlines were backed by ongoing support, which is much appreciated. And I thank Linda Konner, my literary agent, for introducing me to the world of professional writers.

Last but not least, I would like to thank the countless patients and their families who have allowed me the privilege of working with them. They have shared not only their struggles but also the joys that come with overcoming addiction and entering recovery. Being a part of their lives has made me a wiser and better clinician and enriched me as a person. Watching them change as they emerged through the ups and downs of treatment has been the most rewarding experience of my professional life. I shared the journey with them, and as much as I helped them, they helped me. This book is a result of this experience, and I hope it will help others, both people struggling with addiction and their families, to have uplifting journeys into the world of recovery.

NOTES

Introduction

3 When powerful opioids became available: Jane Porter and Hershel Jick, "Addiction Rare in Patients Treated with Narcotics," *New England Journal of Medicine 302*, no. 2 (January 1980): 123, ncbi.nlm.nih.gov/pubmed/7350425.

3 Fast-forward to 2015: International Narcotics Control Board, "Report of the International Narcotics Control Board for 2015," January 2016, incb.org/incb/en/publications/annual-reports/annual-report-2015.html; Rose A. Rudd et al., "Increases in Drug and Opioid-Involved Overdose Deaths—United States, 2010–2015," Morbidity and Mortality Weekly Report, 65 (2016): 1445–52, doi.org/10.15585/mmwr.mm655051e1.

3 In 2016, drug overdoses caused US life expectancy: Kenneth D. Kochanek et al., "Mortality in the United States, 2016," NCHS Data Brief, 293 (December 2017), cdc.gov/nchs/data/databriefs/db293.pdf.

3 about 75 percent of opioid users: Center for Behavioral Health Statistics and Quality, "Results from the 2014 National Survey on Drug Use and Health: Detailed Tables," September 2015, samhsa.gov/data/sites/default/files/NSDUH-DetTabs2014/NSDUH-DetTabs2014.pdf.

4 Opioids create "junkies": Center for Behavioral Health Statistics and Quality, Results from the 2014.

5 more than twenty years into the epidemic: Emanuel Krebs et al., "Cost-Effectiveness of Publicly Funded Treatment of Opioid Use Disorder in California," *Annals of Internal Medicine 168*, no. 1 (2018), doi.org/10.7326/M17-0611; Substance Abuse and Mental Health Services Administration, "National Survey of Substance Abuse Treatment Services (N-SSATS): 2013," 2014, samhsa.gov/data/sites/default/files/2013_N-SSATS_National_Survey_of_Substance_Abuse_Treatment_Services/2013_N-SSATS_National_Survey_of_Substance_Abuse_Treatment_Services.html.

6 up to 90 percent of patients: Substance Abuse and Mental Health Services Administration, "Treatment Episode Data Set (TEDS): 2013. Discharges from Substance Abuse Treatment Services," 2016, samhsa.gov/data/sites/default/files/2013_Treatment_Episode_Data_Set_Discharges_9_14_16.pdf.

6 It is a rare day: Adam Bisaga and Maria A. Sullivan, "Death by Detoxification," *Huffington Post*, August 27, 2013, huffingtonpost.com/adam-bisaga-md/medication-assisted-recovery_b_3824013.html.

Chapter 1: Medical Panacea or National Nightmare?

11 In eastern Ohio, a police officer: CBS News, "Officer Recounts Near-Fatal Contact with Opioid After Traffic Stop," May 17, 2017, cbsnews.com/news/fentanyl-nearly-kills-officer-chris-green-after-drug-arrest-ohio/.

12 Beginning in 2015: Rose A. Rudd et al., "Increases in Drug and Opioid-Involved Overdose Deaths—United States, 2010–2015," Morbidity and Mortality Weekly Report, 65 (2016), 1445–52, doi.org/10.15585/mmwr.mm655051e1.

12 In 2016, the number of deaths: Holly Hedegaard et al., "Drug Overdose Deaths in the United States, 1999–2016," National Center for Health Statistics, 294, (2017), cdc.gov/nchs/products/databriefs/db294.htm; Cancer.net Editorial Board, "Breast Cancer—Metastatic: Statistics," ASCO Cancer.net, accessed December 15, 2017, cancer.net/cancer-types/breast-cancer-metastatic/statistics.

12 Reported fatal overdoses: Hedegaard, Drug Overdose Deaths.

12 More than 42,000 died: Hedegaard, Drug Overdose Deaths.

12 Between 2013 and 2016: Josh Katz, "The First Count of Fentanyl Deaths in 2016: Up 540% in Three Years, New York Times, September 2, 2017, nytimes.com/interactive/2017/09/02/upshot/fentanyl-drug-overdose-deaths.html; National Center for Health Statistics, "Provisional Drug Overdose Death Counts," January 12, 2018, cdc.gov/nchs/nvss/vsrr/drug-overdose-data.htm.

12 In 2009: Leonard J. Paulozzi et al., "Vital Signs: Overdoses of Prescription Opioid Pain Relievers—United States, 1999–2008," Morbidity and Mortality Weekly Report, 60, no. 5, (2011), cdc.gov/mmwr/preview/mmwrhtml/mm6043a4.htm.

12 In 2015: Center for Behavioral Health Statistics and Quality, "Key Substance Use and Mental Health Indicators in the United States: Results from the 2015 National Survey on Drug Use and Health," 2016, samhsa.gov/data/

12 Between 1999 and 2010: Centers for Disease Control and Prevention, "Prescription Painkiller Overdoses: A Growing Epidemic, Especially Among Women," 2013, cdc.gov/vitalsigns/prescriptionpainkilleroverdoses/index.html.

13 In towns hardest hit: Hedegaard, Drug Overdose Deaths

13 In 2015, the Centers for Disease Control: Julie Turkewitz, "The Pills Are Everywhere: How the Opioid Crisis Claims Its Youngest Victims," New York Times, September 20, 2017, nytimes.com/2017/09/20/us/opioid-deaths-children.html.

20 In a seminal experiment: Abraham Wikler, "A Psychodynamic Study of a Patient During Experimental Self-Regulated Re-addiction to Morphine," Psychiatric Quarterly 26, no. 2 (April 1952): 270–93, ncbi.nlm.nih.gov/pubmed/14920640.

25 Since 1939, it has sold: Alcoholics Anonymous, "A.A.'s Big Book, Alcoholics Anonymous, Named by Library of Congress as One of the 'Books That Shaped America,'" press release, July 27, 2012, aa.org/press-releases/en_US/press-releases/aas-big-book-alcoholics-anonymous-named-by-library-of-congress-as-one-of-the-books-that-shaped-america.

28 Less than 10 percent: Substance Abuse and Mental Health Services Administration, "National Survey of Substance Abuse Treatment Services (N-SSATS): 2013. Data on Substance Abuse Treatment Facilities," Substance Abuse and Mental Health Services Administration, 2014.

29 Medications have been shown: Cindy Parks Thomas et al., "Medication-Assisted Treatment With Buprenorphine: Assessing the Evidence," Psychiatric Services 65, no. 2 (2014): 158–70, doi.org/10.1176/appi.ps.201300256; Yih-Ing Hser et al., "Treatment Retention Among Patients

Randomized to Buprenorphine/Naloxone Compared to Methadone in a Multi-site Trial," *Addiction 109,* no. 1 (2014): 79–87, doi.org/10.1111/add.12333; Richard P. Mattick et al., "Buprenorphine Maintenance versus Placebo or Methadone Maintenance for Opioid Dependence," Cochrane Database of Systematic Reviews (February 2014), doi.org/10.1002/14651858.CD002207. pub4; Joshua D. Lee et al., "Comparative Effectiveness of Extended-Release Naltrexone versus Buprenorphine-Naloxone for Opioid Relapse Prevention (X:BOT): A Multicentre, Open-Label, Randomised Controlled Trial," The Lancet (2017), doi.org/10.1016/S0140-6736(17)32812-X; Joshua D. Lee et al., "Extended-Release Naltrexone to Prevent Opioid Relapse in Criminal Justice Offenders," *The New England Journal of Medicine,* 374 (2016): 1232–1242, doi.org/10.1056/ NEJMoa1505409; Evgeny Krupitsky et al., "Injectable Extended-Release Naltrexone for Opioid Dependence: A Double-Blind, Placebo-Controlled, Multicentre Randomised Trial," The Lancet (2011), doi.org/10.1016/S0140-6736(11)60358-9.

Chapter 2: Opioid Use in America: How We Got Here

34 researchers did come to the opinion: David T. Courtwright, *Dark Paradise: A History of Opiate Addiction in America* (Cambridge: Harvard University Press, 1982; President and Fellows of Harvard College, 2001), loc. 1230 of 4538, Kindle.

38 In 1969: Courtwright, *Dark Paradise,* loc. 2242 of 4538, Kindle.

39 "medical" treatments of heroin addiction: H. D. Kleber and C. E. Riordan, "The Treatment of Narcotic Withdrawal: A Historical Review," *Journal of Clinical Psychiatry 43,* no. 6 (1982): 30–34, ncbi.nlm.nih.gov/pubmed/7045089.

40 But overall, the methadone-based treatment: Richard P. Mattick et al., "Buprenorphine Maintenance Versus Placebo or Methadone Maintenance for Opioid Dependence," Cochrane Database of Systematic Reviews (February 2014), doi.org/10.1002/14651858.CD002207. pub4; J. F. Maddux and D. P. Desmond, "Methadone Maintenance and Recovery from Opioid Dependence," *American Journal of Drug and Alcohol Abuse 18,* no. 1 (1992): 63–74.

40 In the mid-1970s: Peter Kerr, "Growth in Heroin Use Ending as City Users Turn to Crack," *New York Times,* September 13, 1986, nytimes.com/1986/09/13/nyregion/growth-in-heroin-use-ending-as-city-users-turn-to-crack.html?pagewanted=all&mcubz=0.

40 By comparison: NYC Health, "Health Department Releases 2016 Drug Overdose Death Data in New York City—1,374 Deaths Confirmed, a 46 Percent Increase From 2015," June 13, 2017, www1.nyc.gov/site/doh/about/press/pr2017/pr048-17.page.

40 By 1984: Substance Abuse and Mental Health Services Administration, "National Survey of Substance Abuse Treatment Services (N-SSATS): 2013," 2014, samhsa.gov/data/sites/default/ files/2013_N-SSATS_National_Survey_of_Substance_Abuse_Treatment_Services/2013_N-SSATS_National_Survey_of_Substance_Abuse_Treatment_Services.html

42 in 1986, and estimated 500,000: Kerr, "Growth in Heroin Use."

42 approximately 5 percent of the population: Center for Behavioral Health Statistics, "2015 National Survey on Drug Use and Health," September 2016, samhsa.gov/data/sites/default/files/ NSDUH-MethodSummDefsHTML-2015/NSDUH-MethodSummDefsHTML-2015/NSDUH-MethodSummDefs-2015.pdf.

43 Within sixteen months: KFF.org, "Global HIV/AIDS Timeline," November 29, 2016, kff.org/ global-health-policy/timeline/global-hivaids-timeline/.

44 Today, just over one million Americans: HIV.gov, "U.S. Statistics: Fast Facts," December 5, 2017, hiv.gov/hiv-basics/overview/data-and-trends/statistics.

44 Close to 2.5 million Americans: Center for Behavioral Health Statistics and Quality, "Key substance use and mental health indicators in the United States: Results from the 2015 National Survey on Drug Use and Health," 2016, samhsa.gov/data/; Substance Abuse and Mental Health Services Administration, National Survey

44 More than forty-two thousand people died: Centers for Disease Control and Prevention, "Opioid Overdose," updated October 23, 2017, cdc.gov/drugoverdose/index.html.

47 the CDC came out with a report: Deborah Dowell et al., "CDC Guideline for Prescribing Opioids for Chronic Pain—United States, 2016," Morbidity and Mortality Weekly Report 65, no. 1 (March 18, 2016): 1–49, doi.org/10.15585/mmwr.rr6501e1.

48 the overall number of patients living with OUD: Yih-Ing Hser et al., "A 33-Year Follow-Up of Narcotics Addicts," Archives of General Psychiatry 58, no. 5 (May 2001): 503–508, ncbi.nlm.nih.gov/pubmed/11343531; Yih-Ing Hser et al., "Long-Term Course of Opioid Addiction," Harvard Review of Psychiatry 23, no. 2 (March–April 2015): 76–89, doi.org/10.1097/HRP.0000000000000052.

48 Only about 3 percent . . . and 40 percent: Alison B. Rapoport and Christopher F. Rowley, "Stretching the Scope—Becoming Frontline Addiction-Medicine Providers," New England Journal of Medicine 377 (2017): 705–707, doi.org/10.1056/NEJMp1706492; Bradley D. Stein et al., "Supply of Buprenorphine Waivered Physicians: The Influence of State Policies," Journal of Substance Abuse Treatment 48, no. 1 (2015): 104–111, doi.org/10.1016/j.jsat.2014.07.010.

49 Overdoses took a dive: Mélina Fatséas and Marc Auriacombe, "Why Buprenorphine Is So Successful in Treating Opiate Addiction in France," Current Psychiatry Reports 9, no. 5 (2007): 358–64, ncbi.nlm.nih.gov/pubmed/17915074.

Chapter 3: Opioid Use Disorder—A Disease Like Any Other?

54 why do nearly 25 percent: Olga A. Vsevolozhskaya and James C. Anthony, "Transitioning from First Drug Use to Dependence Onset: Illustration of a Multiparametric Approach for Comparative Epidemiology," Neuropsychopharmacology 41, no. 3 (February 2016): 869–76, doi.org/10.1038/npp.2015.213.

60 Some of the key behaviors: Adapted from American Psychiatric Association, Diagnostic and Statistical Manual of Mental Disorders (5th ed.) (Arlington, VA: American Psychiatric Publishing, 2013).

68 By simply interacting: Holly Hagan et al., "Reduced Injection Frequency and Increased Entry and Retention in Drug Treatment Associated with Needle-Exchange Participation in Seattle Drug Injectors," Journal of Substance Abuse Treatment 19, no. 3 (October 2000): 247–252, ncbi.nlm.nih.gov/pubmed/11027894.

Chapter 4: Embracing the New Medical Approach to Treating OUD

78 a very high failure rate: Bobby P. Smyth et al., "Lapse and Relapse Following Inpatient Treatment of Opiate Dependence," *Irish Medical Journal* 103, no.6 (June 2010): 176–79; Johan Kakko et al., "1-Year Retention and Social Function after Buprenorphine-Assisted Relapse Prevention Treatment for Heroin Dependence in Sweden: A Randomised, Placebo-Controlled Trial," *Lancet* 361, no. 9358 (February 22, 2003): 662–68, ncbi.nlm.nih.gov/pubmed/12606177.

79 One third of opioid: Shane Darke et al., "Patterns of Nonfatal Heroin Overdose Over a 3-Year Period: Findings From the Australian Treatment Outcome Study," *Journal of Urban Health* 84, no.2 (March 2007): 283–91, doi.org/10.1007/s11524-006-9156-0.

79 Half of heroin: Alexander Caudarella et al., "Non-fatal Overdose as a Risk Factor for Subsequent Fatal Overdose Among People Who Inject Drugs," *Drug and Alcohol Dependence* 162 (May 1, 2016): 51–55, doi.org/10.1016/j.drugalcdep.2016.02.024.

Chapter 5: The Pharmacology of Opioids

97 reducing overdoses by at least half . . . 75 percent of those who start methadone: Shane Darke et al., "Non-fatal Heroin Overdose, Treatment Exposure and Client Characteristics: Findings from the Australian Treatment Outcome Study (ATOS)," *Drug and Alcohol Review* 24, no. 5 (September 2005): 425–32, ncbi.nlm.nih.gov/pubmed/16298837/; Catherine Anne Fullerton et al., "Medication-Assisted Treatment with Methadone: Assessing the Evidence," *Psychiatric Services* 65, no. 2 (2014): 146–57, doi.org/10.1176/appi.ps.201300235; Yih-Ing Hser et al., "Treatment Retention among Patients Randomized to Buprenorphine/Naloxone Compared to Methadone in a Multi-site Trial," *Addiction* 109, no. 1 (2014): 79–87, doi.org/10.1111/add.12333; Richard P. Mattick et al., "Buprenorphine Maintenance versus Placebo or Methadone Maintenance for Opioid Dependence," *Cochrane Database of Systematic Reviews* (2014), doi.org/10.1002/14651858. CD002207.pub4.

98 On average, 50 percent of people on buprenorphine: Cindy Parks Thomas et al., "Medication-Assisted Treatment with Buprenorphine: Assessing the Evidence," *Psychiatric Services* 65, no. 2 (2014): 158–70, doi.org/10.1176/appi.ps.201300256; Yih-Ing Hser, Treatment Retention among Patients; Richard P. Mattick, Buprenorphine Maintenance versus Placebo.

99 Up to 50 percent . . . XR-naltrexone injections: Joshua D. Lee et al., "Comparative Effectiveness of Extended-Release Naltrexone versus Buprenorphine-Naloxone for Opioid Relapse Prevention (X:BOT): A Multicentre, Open-Label, Randomised Controlled Trial," *The Lancet* (2017), doi. org/10.1016/S0140-6736(17)32812-X; Joshua D. Lee et al., "Extended-Release Naltrexone to Prevent Opioid Relapse in Criminal Justice Offenders," *The New England Journal of Medicine* 374 (2016): 1232–1242, doi.org/10.1056/NEJMoa1505409; Evgeny Krupitsky et al., "Injectable Extended-Release Naltrexone for Opioid Dependence: A Double-Blind, Placebo-Controlled, Multicentre Randomised Trial," *The Lancet* (2011), doi.org/10.1016/S0140-6736(11)60358-9.

99 About 30 to 40 percent . . . actively using opioids: Joshua D. Lee, Comparative Effectiveness of.

Chapter 7: When Treating OUD Becomes a Challenge

126 However, initial experience with: Erin Kelty and G. Hulse, "A Retrospective Cohort Study of Obstetric Outcomes in Opioid-Dependent Women Treated with Implant Naltrexone, Oral Methadone or Sublingual Buprenorphine, and Non-Dependent Controls," *Drugs* 77, no. 11 (July 2017): 1199–1210, doi.org/10.1007/s40265-017-0762-9.

126 Methadone used to be the gold standard: S. L. Klaman, "Treating Women Who Are Pregnant and Parenting for Opioid Use Disorder and the Concurrent Care of Their Infants and Children: Literature Review to Support National Guidance," *Journal of Addiction Medicine* 11, no.3 (May/June 2017): 178–90, doi.org/10.1097/ADM.0000000000000308.

139 In 2016: Deborah Dowell et al., "CDC Guideline for Prescribing Opioids for Chronic Pain—United States, 2016," Morbidity and Mortality Weekly Report 65, no. 1 (March 18, 2016): 1–49, doi.org/10.15585/mmwr.rr6501e1.

141 Another issue is that: Theodore J. Cicero et al., "Correspondence: Effect of Abuse-Deterrent Formulation of OxyContin," *New England Journal of Medicine* 367 (2012): 187–89, doi.org/10.1056/NEJMc1204141.

141 Half of all patients: L. Dhingra et al., "Epidemiology of Pain Among Outpatients in Methadone Maintenance Treatment Programs," *Drug and Alcohol Dependence* 128, no. 1–2 (February 1, 2013): 161–65, doi.org/10.1016/j.drugalcdep.2012.08.003.

Chapter 8: How to Encourage Your Loved One to Get Help—and How to Help Yourself

154 Motivational interviewing is a strategy: William R. Miller and Stephen Rollnick, *Motivational Interviewing: Helping People Change,* 3rd ed. (New York: Guilford Press, 2012).

164 people with a history of overdose: Shane Darke et al., "Non-fatal Heroin Overdose, Treatment Exposure and Client Characteristics: Findings from the Australian Treatment Outcome Study (ATOS)," *Drug and Alcohol Review 24, n. 5* (September 2005): 425–32, ncbi.nlm.nih.gov/pubmed/16298837/.

171 CRAFT is outlined: Robert J. Meyers and Brenda L. Wolfe, *Get Your Loved One Sober: Alternatives to Nagging, Pleading, and Threatening* (Center City, MN: Hazelden, 2003).

Chapter 9: Finding the Right Treatment

177 2.4 million people suffering from: Center for Behavioral Health Statistics and Quality, "Key Substance Use and Mental Health Indicators in the United States: Results from the 2015 National Survey on Drug Use and Health," 2016, samhsa.gov/data/.

Chapter 10: How to Support Your Loved One in Treatment and Recovery

199 In one study: Adam R. Winstock et al., "'Should I stay or should I go?' Coming off methadone and buprenorphine treatment," *International Journal of Drug Policy* 22, no. 1 (2011): 77–81.

Epilogue: Overdoses as Missed Opportunities

253 About one in twenty: Shane Darke et al., "The ratio of non-fatal to fatal overdose," *Addiction* 98 (2003): 1169–70; Albert Espelt et al., "Lethality of Opioid Overdose in a Community Cohort of Young Heroin Users," *European Addiction Research* 21, no. 6 (2015): 300–306, doi.org/10.1159/000377626.

253 When opioid overdose victims . . . buprenorphine: Gail D'Onofrio et al., "Emergency Department–Initiated Buprenorphine/Naloxone Treatment for Opioid Dependence: A Randomized Clinical Trial," *Journal of the American Medical Association* 313, no. 16 (2015): 1636–44, doi.org/10.1001/jama.2015.3474.

254 In just three short years: Josh Katz, "The First Count of Fentanyl Deaths in 2016: Up 540% in Three Years," *New York Times,* September 2, 2017, nytimes.com/interactive/2017/09/02/upshot/fentanyl-drug-overdose-deaths.html.

INDEX

and treatment for pain, 143
See also XR-naltrexone
Narcan. *See* naloxone
Narcotics Anonymous (NA), 22, 210, 225, 241
neonatal abstinence syndrome (NAS), 111, 129–30
Nicole's story, 61–62, 111–12, 197–98
noradrenaline, 57
Nyswander, Marie, 39

O

opiates
overview, 15
   heroin, 5, 34–35, 38–39, 49, 90–93, 117–18
   morphine, 15, 17, 33–34
   opioids
   overview, 7, 15–16
   campaign to de-stigmatize addiction, 3
   carfentanil, 16
   emotion suppression, 74, 180
   and human body, 86, 87–90
   methamphetamine-opioid combinations, 50, 254–55
oxycodone, 111–12, 174–75, 177
   as painkillers vs. nonmedical use, 3–4
   as treatment for opioid addiction, 36–37
   See also cycles of opioid use in America; fentanyl; methadone; opiates
opioid addiction. See opioid use disorder
opioid addiction treatment, 174–93
   abstinence-based programs, 27–28
   fear of, 177–78
   early initiation of, 61
   as first step on a long road, 2

inadequacy of current system, xii–xiii, 6–7
in late 1800s–early 1920s, 35–37
methadone clinics, 39–40
OTPs, 37, 40, 93, 100, 108, 183, 257, 260
personality disorder approach, x–xi, 21–22
See also medication-assisted treatment; OUD treatment/ overdose prevention medications
opioid crisis, 3–4, 12, 253–56. See also social context of addiction crisis
opioid-free by choice, 219–51
   overview, 219–20
   alternatives to quitting, 224–25
   conflicting voices exercise, 222–24
   first days and weeks, 237–45
   next months and years, 246–51
   understanding why you use, 222
   your hopes, 221–22
   your problems and strengths, 220–21
   See also recovery
opioid intoxication signs, 158
opioid receptor system
   overview, 86–87, 89–90
   and buprenorphine, 95, 96
   and methadone, 93–94
   and naltrexone, 96–97
opioid treatment programs (OTPs), 37, 40, 93, 100, 108, 183, 257, 260
opioid treatment system, 179
opioid use disorder (OUD), 51–67
   overview, 5, 53–54, 104–5
   and brain chemistry, 52–53, 56–57
   as chronic condition, 48, 53–54, 62–63, 76, 198–99, 246–51
   development of, 17–20
   diagnostic standards, 59–61, 82–83
   doctor shortage, 48–49

ABOUT THE AUTHORS

Adam Bisaga, MD, is an addiction psychiatrist, clinician, researcher, and professor of psychiatry at Columbia University. He conducts research on new treatments for opioid addiction and oversees a national program that mentors physicians treating opioid addictions. He is a UN expert involved in international addiction training and program development, and he recently co-edited the UN/WHO "International Standards for the Treatment of Drug Use Disorders."

Karen Chernyaev is a writer and editor with more than thirty years' experience in publishing. She has worked on dozens of books on addiction treatment, recovery, and related topics.